Chapter 1

Once upon a time there was a little town called Health-land kingdom, located right off the big super MD highway leading to the great cure-all metropolis. In this town lived vitamins, minerals, herbs, humans, and other nutrients.

The town's main goal was to keep all of its citizens healthy because anyone that   they failed to keep healthy would have to face terrible traffic jams on the super MD highway leading to the great cure-all metropolis.

Jim-Niacin (vitamin B-3). Jim-Niacin doesn't stand alone; he is a member of the very powerful B vitamin family. In Health-land Jim-Niacin's job is essential to promote life and good health. He regulates the metabolism and assists in other body processes, even though he is needed in small amounts compared to proteins and carbohydrates.

As a coenzyme Jim-Niacin works
to make sure the human body
functions as it should. There are two
major types of vitamins: the water
soluble and the oil soluble. Jim-Niacin
belongs to the water-soluble type
vitamins, therefore his doses
must be replaced everyday because
the human body doesn't store his
doses like the oil soluble type.

Since Jim-Niacin is only one
member of the very powerful B
vitamin family he shouldn't work
alone; he should be balanced with
other B vitamin members. Jim-Niacin
is not a bad or evil fellow, but he does
have a bad reputation.

Humans are afraid of Jim-Niacin
and rightly so because in too high
doses he may damage the liver, or in
too low doses he does no good. But,
that is not the only reason human
fear Jim-Niacin. Jim-Niacin deals with
circulation and the skin, and he will
heat the skin up like it is on fire and
turn it as red as a beet.
When this happens to a human

for the first time, it will scare some humans half to death, but don't be put off, the flushing of the skin is normal when dealing with Jim-Niacin. It's not pretty or pleasant but that is how Jim-Niacin unclogs the capillaries and small blood vessels throughout the body.

Captain Fredrico (human). Orry Fredrico is one of many humans that Was born and raised in Health-land Kingdom. Orry Fredrico is a Carpenter by trade, but as long as he Could remember he loved the sea. As a small child he would stand by The ocean for hours just staring out to Sea.

As a teenager he would try to Hop aboard any boat going salt water Fishing. During his senior year in high School he went on one of those deep Sea fishing cruises that goes out for Four or five hours at a time. On this Cruises he met Jan Flemmings. Jan Also loved the sea and they instantly Became attracted to each other.

Within days Jim started dating Jan.

VC (vitamin C). VC also belongs
To the water-soluble type of vitamin.
VC   is truly a heavyweight among
Vitamins. VC is known as a very
Power antioxidant. He is a mighty
Human body protector. He protects
the human body against harmful
effects of pollution.   He helps to
prevent cancer.   He helps to lower
cholesterol and other protection
functions.

Scurvy is a disease that moves
in when there is a deficiency in
vitamin C protection. Years ago,
passengers on ships on long voyages
without fresh fruits and vegetables
had a problem dealing with scurvy.

Jan Flemmings (human). Jan
is a Health-land Kingdom toy
soldier's brat. Just like Captain
Fredrico she has always loved the

sea. She was mostly unanchored until she met her   soul mate Orry Fredrico. At first she thought he loved the sea too much and would not be a good provider, but his dreamy bedroom eyes soon won her over.

VE (vitamin E). VE belongs to the oil soluble type of vitamin. VE is another mighty antioxidant. VE is very important in fighting cancer and cardiovascular disease. Vitamin E is a giant in so many ways. VE is a natural blood thinner. He promotes good blood circulation, he promotes healthy skin, healthy hair, and so many other healthy body functions. Vitamin E actually belongs to a family of eight but falls into two major groups. These two groups are tocopherols and tocotrienols. It is the alpha-tocopherols form that is the most potent. That is the group VE belongs to.

John-Pyridoxine (vitamin B-6). John-Pyridoxine like his cousin Jim-Niacin is a member of the very powerful B vitamin family. The fact is John-Pyridoxine is involved in more bodily functions than any other single nutrient. John-Pyridoxine deals with both the mental and physical health.

He deals with water retention, sodium and potassium balance, and fights hard against allergies, arthritis, asthma, carpal tunnel syndrome, and on and on. Just like his cousin Jim-Niacin, John-Pyridoxine shouldn't fight alone; he should be balanced with other members of the mighty B vitamin family.

Mister Disease. Mister and his family   showed up one day in Health-land Kingdom. No one seems to know where he came from. All anyone knows is he is mean and evil. He has no friends and is known to attack humans sometimes without provocation.

He has no conscience and will attack anyone that is weak and helpless. The town and kingdom has tried to keep him out, but somehow he always sneaks back in. Our vitamins, minerals, herbs and others nutrient citizens have done a good job fighting him off, but Mister Disease is a very, very tough customer.

       Jim-Niacin and the other nutrient protectors of Health-land Kingdom were joyfully patting themselves on the back because they were doing a good job protecting the city's population from Mister Disease and his cohorts. Jim-Niacin decided to telephone his cousin John-Pyridoxine. Jim could hear the phone making its fourth ring.

"Hello," said John-Pyridoxine.
" This is Jim-Niacin, I decided to give you a call and touch base on a matter that I've been tossing around

in my mind lately."
"Tell me about it," said John-Pyridoxine.

"Well, I've been thinking that all of the vitamins, minerals, humans, herbs, and other nutrient citizens should get together and have a big town hall meeting. What do you think."

"I think it is a very good idea," said john-Pyridoxine.
" Good, then it's a go, I'm going to start right away making plans," said Jim-Niacin. "John you take care now, I'll talk to you later."
" Bye," said John-Pyridoxine.

Chapter 2

        Orry Fredrico and Jan Flemmings got married after a one year engagement. Orry got an associate degree in carpentry from the local technical college. Twenty five years later Orry and Jan are now the parents of a seventeen-year-old son Rob, and a fifteen-year-old daughter Melinda.

Almost everyone calls Orry   by his nickname Captain Fredrico after he bought his first boat about fifteen years ago. The boat was a fourteen footer with a big Mercury motor. Captain Fredrico now operates his own contracting business.

It is almost six o'clock p.m. when Captain Fredrico lets himself in the carport door which opens directly into the kitchen. He found his wife Jan bending over checking her meat loaf in the oven.

"Hello dear," said Captain Fredrico in a somewhat tired voice. " Hello Orry, how did your day " Pretty good, but my right wrist that's been bothering me the last couple of weeks seems to be getting worse, especially at night after I fall asleep.   Sometimes I wake up with a numb tingling in my right hand. It feels like somebody is sticking pins in my hands."

"Orry, I think you need to check with one of the vitamin citizens. That sounds like something John-pyridoxine might be able to help you with."

"I think you are right dear, I will give him a call in a few days.

After Marrying Orry, Jan Fredrico decided to postpone a career of her own. Becoming a full time housewife and mother was very fulfilling to Jan. She even took on the   awesome job of home schooling her kids.

VC (vitamin c) enjoys his job in Health-land Kingdom taking care of its citizens. He has a very good reputation. Humans were using him probably more than any other vitamin. Being one of the most powerful antioxidants, he was in great demand these days.

In fact, he was being used to fortify many of today's foods. He thought the town hall meeting was a great idea. Why didn't he think of it? The vitamins and other nutrients were doing a good job fighting off Mister Disease, but he knew that they couldn't let their guards down, ever.

Just like VC, VE (vitamin E) is another very powerful antioxidant but of the oil soluble type. VE is probably in even greater demand these days than VC. With so many humans becoming diabetics these days, VE with his natural blood thinning power is a real workhorse. VE is also looking forward to the big town hall meeting coming up soon.

On this Monday morning John-Pyridoxine was kicking back at his office when the phone ring.

" Hello," said John-Pyridoxine.
" May I speak to John-Pyridoxine?" said the voice on the line.

"This is he," said John-Pyridoxine.
" I'm Captain Fredrico and I've been told you may be able to help me concerning an ailment. I believe I have a case of carpal tunnel syndrome."

"You have the right vitamin, that is one of my many areas of expertise."
" Then you will be able to help me," said Captain Fredrico.

"Hold on a minute, I didn't say that. Let me explain the situation here, then I can tell you what I may be able to do. Listen Captain, I'm going to explain what I do, and it should take care of your problem, but then it may not. If I can't cure it, then I recommend you take the super MD highway to the cure all metropolis."

"I understand," said Captain Fredrico.

" Now, first off," said John-Pyridoxine, "my maximum dose is 300 mg. per day, that way I will not damage any nerves. In most cases 100 mg. of my dose will cure the problem. The golden rule with taking any nutrients is don't take more than the recommended dose, because too much of anything may cause damage, and never take nutrients on an empty stomach. So, Captain if you understood everything I said, come by as soon as possible. We have a walk in policy."

"Thank you sir, I should be there within the hour."

Mister Disease is very upset with himself for being unable to do more damage in Health-land Kingdom. He feels he should be able to bring in more of his friends like cancer, AIDS, and even some of his very old friends like the black plague.

He was getting fed up with those damn vitamins, minerals, herbs, and other nutrients. The thing about those nutrients is they are keeping him from getting a foothold in Health-land Kingdom. He feels that if he could just get a foothold he would be able to start an epidemic.

Mister Disease decided that he would just have to work harder. Sooner or later those humans are going to think that they are safe and slack up on utilizing the nutrients. That is the time he plans to throw his best punch. He feels that if his friend AIDS just keeps up the pressure, he has the best shot at causing an epidemic.

Most humans don't know Jim-Niacin and many of those that do tend to fear and avoid him. As one of the smallest members of the powerful B vitamin family, being unknown is about to change. The reason is Jim-

Niacin along with his cousin John-Pyridoxine are the ones that called for and organized the town hall meeting coming up in a few weeks. The whole thing was originally Jim-Niacin's idea.

Since then Jim has invited the town fathers and secured all of the permits needed to stage such an event. Jim has contacted other town nutrients and humans, many of them had never heard of him, or knew who he was.

Chapter 3

Captain Fredrico had lived in Health-land Kingdom all of his life and he loved this town. Captain Fredrico got an invitation from Jim-Niacin to attend the town hall meeting coming up in a few weeks.

Captain Fredrico had heard the name Jim-Niacin before and even knew he was a member of the mighty

B vitamin family, but that was about all he knew about Jim-Niacin. He didn't know what kind of work or anything else Jim-Niacin did.

Captain Fredrico had heard that the vitamins and other nutrients citizens had become concerned about the health of Health-land Kingdom. The main work our nutrient citizens do is protect our human population from characters like Mister Disease and his friends.

The nutrients knew that cancer and AIDS had almost destroyed a few other towns in the Kingdom. The town hall meeting got Captain Fredrico to thinking. The mayoral election will be coming up in about a year. Captain Fredrico decided that he was going to throw his hat in the ring. Of course he would have to talk it over with his wife Jan first.

After putting in a hard day's work, on his drive home Captain Fredrico thought about the pesky dry skin that had been plaguing him for years. It has slowly become more and more of a problem as time past.

Now it has become a real nuisance. It has come to the point that he has to lotion down almost his whole body every time he takes a shower.
He feels that is unmanly, only women like to lotion their bodies. He has tried everything, but to no avail.

He had even got on the crowded super MD highway and went to the cure all metropolis, but still to no avail. At the cure all metropolis all they did was to prescribe an extremely expensive body cream that did little better than over the counter creams.

He felt truly at his wits end.
There didn't seem to be any hope, he would just have to accept his miserable fate. As Captain Fredrico let himself in the carport door, Jan was making a salad.
" Hello, dear," said the Captain in a husky sexy voice.

"Hello, sweetheart," said Jan in a wooing voice as she dropped everything and rushed over and planted a seductive kiss on her husband's left cheek.

"Now, you go ahead and clean up, dinner will be ready in a few minutes. By the way Rob complained about a bout of indigestion after lunch."

"Did you check with Mr. Blue Page?" said the Captain.
" Yes, he gave me the names of several nutrients that work in that area. The two nutrients that I decided to use were Stewart-Ginger Root and Henry-Acidolphilus. Each one of them gave me heavy doses to give Rob as needed."

"Good, now let me go ahead and wash up, then you can tell me all about it later." After the Captain and all of the family had sat down to dinner and the blessing was said, the Captain revisited the subject of Rob's indigestion.

"How is your stomach feeling now, Rob," said the Captain.
" It's fine now, dad, since Mom had a couple of the nutrients treat it."
" I wasn't sure what to do until after my talk with Mr. Blue Page," said Jan.

"Mr. Blue Page gave me the names of several nutrients that work in the area of indigestion. These are the names that Mr. Blue Page gave me that deal with indigestion: Stewart-Ginger Root, Calvin-Fenugreek, Bonnie-Papaya, Henry-Acidophilus, and Sammy-Oat bran tablets.

He also stressed that they did their work with either tablets or capsules."

"Excuse me for changing the subject, I have a very important announcement to make," said the captain.

"Jan, the mayoral election is

coming up in about a year and I would like to know if you have any objections to me throwing my hat into the ring."

"Gee, I don't know? I've never thought about being a politician's wife. Do you think you can win?"
"Dad, I love it, I think it is a great idea," said Melinda.
"Me too," said Rob.

"I can't guarantee you I will win, but I believe if I get out there and shake enough hands I'll have a very good shot."
" Dad, I'll campaign for you," said Melinda.

"Honey, If you really want to run, then count me in as your number one supporter," said Jan.
"Then it's all settled You are looking at the next mayor of Health-land Kingdom."

Ever since John-Pyridoxine had agreed to help his cousin Jim-Niacin organize the big town hall meeting coming up soon, he had stayed busy calling and talking to the citizens of Health-land Kingdom.

Chapter 4

Mr. Disease was aware of the big town hall meeting coming up in a few days, and he definitely was not pleased about what he was hearing. The word was they were going to try to get rid of him. Mr. Disease was not going to let that deter him, that had been tried before with his ancestors all throughout history.

Sure, the discovery of DDT, penicillin, and modern antibiotics had given his family some big setbacks, but some of his old friends like tuberculosis were beginning to make a comeback, and the new kid on the block, AIDS, was really beginning to raise hell.

Mr. Disease felt that as far as he was concerned, let them have all of the town hall meetings they want to, it was not going to put him out of business.

Mr. Disease watches the super MD highway often and as far as he could tell it was becoming even more crowded each day. Even at the big super cure all metropolis they haven't been able to get rid of his best friend Mr. Cancer. Mr. Cancer is still doing an awful lot of damage.

On this Monday morning Jan Fredrico   sure didn't want to battle the traffic jams on the super MD highway going to the cure all metropolis. It was just one of those days, Her daughter was down with a cold and she herself was dealing with a slight kidney infection.

She didn't know? Maybe it was something she ate that was causing her back a slight ache in the area of her kidney. She knew that it would save her a lot of money and time if she called Mr. Blue Page and found out which vitamins, minerals, herbs, or other nutrients that specialized in the areas of their ailments.

Jan decided to give the nutrients twenty-four hours to do their work, then if there was no obvious improvement she would get on the crowded super MD highway to the cure all metropolis. Jan dialed Mr. Blue Page. The voice on the line said, " You have reached Mr. Blue Page directory."
"Mr. Blue Page, this is Jan Fredrico.   My daughter has a cold and my kidneys have a slight ache. I would like for you to give me the names of the nutrients that specialize in the areas of our illness."

"Very well, madam. In the area of the   kidneys, the association of VC and Cranberry handle that, and in the area of colds and flu, the association of Garlic, Echinacea, and Golden Seal handle that. Will that be all, madam?"

"Yes sir, and thank you very

much," said Jan. Taking advantage of their-walk in policy, Jan didn't have to wait long before she was able to see VC, the very powerful vitamin C antioxidant.

"Mrs. Fredrico," said VC, " We give our doses in mostly tablet form. I am of the water soluble type, the body does not store my doses. Taking too much of my dose is washed out with the urine. But, taking too much of my dose also may cause diarrhea or stomach soreness in some humans.

Rule number one for dealing with your kidney problem is to keep drinking lots of water, then take 2000 mg. of vitamin C tablets three or four times a day after a meal, also take 2000 mg. of cranberry fruit capsules three of four times a day after a meal. That should take care of your problem, Mrs. Fredrico."

Jan next proceeded to take her daughter by the association of Garlic, Echinacea, and Golden Seal to take care of her cold. After a short wait Jan and her daughter were lead in to see Hannah-Garlic.

Hannah-Garlic came from one of the most powerful and popular of all herb families. Even   the Roman army would not go into battle without a member of the garlic family coming along.

Hannah-Garlic instructed Jan to give Melinda throat lozenges if needed, then give her a dose of about 1400 mg. of odor controlled garlic, three or four times a day after a meal, also give her a 1500 mg. dose of combination echinacea-golden seal three or four times a day after a meal.

"You should see some obvious improvement in twenty four hours; if not take the super MD highway to the cure all metropolis.

"It is also helpful to take heavy doses of vitamin C after a meal at the beginning of a cold. But, only at the beginning of a cold, because if

congestion sets in, vitamin C tends
to make it worse. Warning: Never
take vitamin C or others nutrients on
an empty stomach," she said.
After thoroughly going over
everything, Hannah-Garlic said, "
That is it, Mrs. Fredrico, do you
understand all of my instructions?"

"Yes, Herb Garlic and thank you
very much." While driving home Jan
reminded herself to do her neck
exercises when she got home. It has
been quite awhile since stress has
caused her neck to tense up, but she
Decided that she would go ahead
and do the exercises anyway.

Jan believed that feeling stress is
a normal part of life. The better one
learns how to deal with life's
frustrations the better one will be able
to cope with stress. Stress affects
people in many different ways. It
may affect some in physical ways
such as headaches, neck aches,
shoulder aches, etc.

To deal with physical aches it is

helpful to do these exercises. These exercises are done sitting on the side of the bed. Sit on the side of the bed with feet apart flat on the floor for balance. With both hands rolled into a fist, place them thumbs inward down on the bed several inches from the body on each side.

Start the first exercise by twisting the neck and entire upper body counter-clockwise as far as possible, then twist the neck and entire upper body clockwise as far as possible. Do these exercises in sets of one hundred as many times as one desires.

Start the second exercise by leaning the head as far as possible on the right shoulder, then lean the head as far as possible on the left shoulder. Do these exercises in sets of one hundred as many times as one desires.

Start the third exercise by leaning the chin as far as possible down on the chest, then lift the head backward as far as possible. Do these exercises in sets of one hundred as many times as one desires.

Chapter 5

On the morning of the big town hall meeting, Jim-Niacin followed his daily routine of taking care of the citizens of Health-land Kingdom. Jim-Niacin tried to take care of all loose ends concerning the town hall meeting by making a lot of last minute phone calls. He rehearsed the program with his cousin B-12 who would be the moderator for tonight's town hall meeting.

At seven o'clock p.m. sharp Jim-Niacin arrived at the local high school gymnasium, the location of tonight's town hall meeting. The meeting was scheduled to start at eight o'clock p.m. There were several satellite trucks already in place when he arrived. There were the local radio and TV crews as well as reporters from the big super cure all metropolis.

Arriving at the high school was familiar territory for Captain Fredrico. He had walked at the high school track three or more times a week for several years. The high school track was a popular walking place for the citizens of Health-land Kingdom. Captain Fredrico felt that walking or some type of physical fitness program is a must to maintain good health.

It is a fact that one in good physical condition has almost a ten times better chance of surviving a heart attack, stroke, or any ailment. Also, physical activity plays a big role in controlling diabetes. A big help with diabetes is controlling what one eats. Most humans can control diabetes by cutting way back on starches and sweets and taking a chromium picolinate at each meal.

One needs to eat less meat and include more peas, beans, fresh fruits, and raw vegetables. One needs to include at least one raw fruit or vegetable at each meal because cooking and microwaving food destroys all enzymes and most vitamins.

Enzymes are involved in almost every bodily function, especially the digestive process. Enzymes are mostly divided into two groups: digestive enzymes and metabolic enzymes. The digestive enzymes break down food enabling the body to function properly.

The human body manufactures a limited supply of enzymes, but in order to prevent indigestion and other digestive problems one should get as many enzymes as possible from raw food. Otherwise, the body's limited supply becomes depleted.

Jim could see that there was going to be a very big turnout for tonight's event. It seemed like his hard work on getting the word out had paid off. Several tables were set up at one end of the gymnasium to try to accommodate as many as possible on the big panel of vitamins, minerals, humans, herbs, and other nutrients.

Everyone were handed a program as they filed into the gymnasium. It read that, "We will not be able to accommodate everyone due to the time it would take. The moderator will ask all questions, but he will take a few written questions from the audience." At exactly eight p.m. sharp B-12 (vitamin B-12) strode up to the podium.

"Greetings, my fellow vitamins, minerals, humans, herbs, and other nutrients, I'm B-12 your moderator for tonight's town hall meeting," he said. "First I would like to welcome our town's fathers, celebrities, and all other dignitaries to this town hall meeting. Now, I would like to thank the vitamin that made it all happen. He is truly another unsung hero. Many of you here tonight probably have never heard of him, but all of the while he has been out there everyday doing his job. He is one of the lesser known members of the powerful B vitamin family. I am proud to say this truly unsung hero is my first cousin Jim-Niacin (vitamin B-3). Stand up, Jim."

"Thank you, thank you, thank you," said Jim-Niacin as he stood and the audience loudly applauded. "Now," said B-12, "before we get into questions and answers we are going to let several members on our panel down here give their name and vocation. We will start with me. I'm B-12 (vitamin B-12). One of my many jobs is to assure proper digestion and the absorption of food."

"I'm Jane-Ginkgo Biloba. I'm a very well known herb. I'm mostly Known for improving memory." "I'm Sammy-Oat Bran Tablets. I'm known for my fiber. Fiber does so many things, for now I will mention just two, I lower the blood cholesterol and help stabilize blood sugar."

"I'm Eddie-calcium. I'm a mineral and I do many things. I'm most needed for strong bones and teeth

and to help lower blood pressure."
"I'm Mary-Magnesium. I'm a mineral and of the many things that I do, enzyme activity is most vital. I also assist calcium and potassium uptake."

"I'm Sue-Chromium. I'm a mineral and of the many things that I do, maintaining stable blood sugar levels is most vital."
"I'm VA (vitamin A). I'm a vitamin and lesser known antioxidant. My main job is protecting the eyes and some skin problems."
"I'm Dee Dee (vitamin D). I'm a vitamin, and I'm needed for the absorption of calcium and phosphorus."

"I'm Ned-Zinc. I'm a mineral and of the many things that I do, keeping the prostate gland healthy is most vital."

"I'm Kenny-Saw Pametto. I'm an herb, my main job is to prevent the enlargement of the prostate gland."
"I'm Gina-Evening Primrose Oil.

I'm an essential fatty acid. I'm a necessity that cannot be made by the human body. I do many things, but improving the skin is my favorite."

"I'm Patty-Potassium. I'm a mineral. Of my many jobs I will name just a few. I help maintain a healthy nervous system and regulate heart rhythm, also I help control the body's water balance."

"I'm Hannah-Garlic. I'm an herb. I detoxify and protect the body against infections. I help lower blood pressure, aid circulation and perform many other functions."

"I'm Henry-Acidophilus. I'm a friendly bacteria. My main job is to aid digestion."

"I'm Bonnie-Papaya. I'm an herb. I aid digestion. I'm good for heartburn, indigestion, and bowel disorders."

"I'm Brad-Cranberry Fruit. I'm an herb. I'm helpful for fighting infections of the urinary track."

"I'm Stewart-Ginger Root. I'm an herb. I do many things, but cleaning the colon, reducing spasms, and stomach cramps is my favorite."

"I'm Calvin-Fenugreek. I'm good for the stomach, intestines, eyes, asthma, sinus, inflammation, and lung disorders. I also increase sexual desire."

"I'm Edna-Echinacea. I'm an herb. I have anti viral properties and I help boost the immune system. I'm very helpful against colds and flu."
"I'm Gene-Golden Seal. I'm an herb. I act as an antibiotic, and have anti-inflammatory and antibacterial properties."

I'm David-Dandelion root. I am an herb. I help cleanse the blood stream and liver and increase the production of bile. I'm used as a diuretic. I help reduce uric acid and improve functioning of the stomach and other vital organs.

"That is the last introduction we will have time for," said B-12. "Now, I will ask the panel a few written questions given to me from the audience, but first let me explain our role here. Number one is we try to be the first line of defense on protecting Health-land Kingdom from Mr. Disease and his cohorts.

"We have some citizens who don't believe in us and won't use our services. The next thing is we don't try to be everything to everybody, our services and abilities are limited.

We encourage anyone that has doubts or don't believe in us to take the super MD highway to the cure all metropolis. Still, there is a lot we can do to keep Mr. Disease and his friends from gaining a foothold here in Health-land Kingdom.

"Very important: When taking the super MD highway to the cure all metropolis, make sure you tell them which of our services you are maintaining.

"Now, when I ask a question to the panel, please let those that specialize in that particular area of expertise answer the question. Time will not allow me to ask but only a few questions. My first question to the panel is what can we do to combat prostate disease?" he asked.
"I'm Ned-Zinc, and I recommend 50 mg. of zinc per day."

"I'm Larry-Pumpkin Seed Oil, and I recommend 1000 mg. of pumpkin seed oil per day."
"I'm Kenny-Saw Pametto, and I recommend 160 mg. of saw pametto extract twice per day."
"I'm VE (vitamin E), and I recommend 1000 I.U. of vitamin E per day."
"I'm Jim-Niacin, and I recommend my maintenance dose of 250 mg. of niacin per day."
"Is there anyone else?" said B-12. "So, that gives us five weapons to fight prostate disease, and I'm pretty darn sure that anyone that

arms themselves with these weapons will be able to keep Mr. prostate disease away for a very long time, if not forever. My next question to the panel is what can we do to deal with diabetes disease?"

"I'm Sue-Chromium, and I recommend 200 mg. of chromium picolinate three times a day at meal time. I also would like to elaborate a little on this terrible disease.

"Diet plays a   major role in controlling this terrible disease. Everyone with this disease should be able to home check his blood sugar level and keep it under control. But, controlling blood sugar is not the only problem diabetics face.

"There are problems with the eyes, blood circulation, and many others. There is a problem with nerve damage (neuropathy) especially in the lower extremities," she concluded.

"I'm VE (vitamin E), and I recommend 1000 I.U. of vitamin E

per day. Being a natural blood thinner makes me a great asset to a diabetic."

"I'm Jim-Niacin, and I recommend my maintenance dose of 250 mg. of niacin once per day for one not showing any diabetic symptoms. On the other hand, for anyone experiencing the symptoms of diabetes, especially numbness in the lower extremities I recommend my unclogging dose of 250 mg. of niacin twice per day.

"Too high of a dose of niacin can cause liver damage and high blood sugar levels, but too low of a dose does no good. The 500 mg. maximum dose per day seems to be just enough to be effective.

"There have been many lower extremities cut off because of diabetes, but I truly believe that if they had only given Jim-Niacin a chance I would have saved some of those limbs."

"Is there anyone else?" said B-12. "There it is folks, three powerful weapons to deal with this scourge diabetes. Now, for the final question of the evening, the question is what can we do to prevent extremely dry skin?"

"I'm Gina-Evening Primrose Oil, I'm an essential fatty acid and I'm one of the good oils that the body needs for beautiful skin. I recommend 1000-3000 mg. of evening primrose oil per day."

"I'm Jim-Niacin. In my view problems with dry skin, toe nail funguses, dandruff, and other skin problems is almost always a problem with blood circulation especially in the capillaries and small blood vessels.

"For extremely dry skin I recommend my unclogging dose of 250 mg. twice per day after a meal until the extremely dry skin condition has been cured, then throttle down to 250 mg. once a day for maintenance. But, be aware, most humans fear me, and for good reason, because my doses are no Sunday picnic or stroll through the park. My doses may heat up your skin like it is on fire and turn it as red as a beet.

"This flushing process is unpredictable, sometimes it will not happen at all, then other times it will last anywhere from five minutes to thirty minutes. It may not be pleasant, but it is my only way of unclogging the capillaries and small blood vessels," said Jim-Niacin.

"Is there anyone else?" said B-12. "What more could one ask for; those were two of the most powerful remedies that I ever heard of in dealing with a pesky humiliating dry skin condition.

"Remember, a dry skin problem is not something to be taken lightly, because you can see what is happening to the outer skin, but what's taking place inside with the vital organs could be a lot worse. "Citizens of Health-land

Kingdom, that will end our town hall meeting for tonight, I would like to thank everyone for coming. Have a safe drive home," he said.

Chapter 6

Captain Fredrico was very impressed with the town hall meeting, especially learning how to deal with his long time dry skin problem and toe nail fungus. It had got to the point that he hated to take a shower.

It was bad enough struggling through the warmer months of the year, but the approach of winter was almost terrifying because a dry skin problem becomes much worse during the winter months. Much of the time during the winter he had to resort to what is called a bird bath by washing only his arm pits and private area. He had tried all kinds of oils, both internal and external. He had traveled on the super MD highway to the cure all metropolis, but all to no avail. Since the town hall meeting he had started off on Jim-Niacin's unclogging dose of 250 mg. of niacin twice a day after a meal.

The resulting benefits were obvious within a couple of days. Within days the treatment was so effective that the captain could barely wait to jump into the shower for the slightest reason. Also, within days his toe nails had started clearing and should be completely clear within a few months.

Also, in a few months the mayoral election will be taking place. Captain Fredrico felt very good about his chances of winning. According to the latest poll he had a four point lead.

That night as he and Jan were setting in the den watching TV, Captain Fredrico said, "You know, Jan, if I do become mayor of Health-land Kingdom I'm going to recognize Jim-Niacin by declaring a Jim-Niacin day."

"I know, dear, how much you love Jim-Niacin. He made it possible for you to be able to take regular showers again without you having to lotion down almost your whole body."
"I don't care how much he is feared and misunderstood," said the Captain. "As far as I'm concerned Jim-Niacin is a miracle vitamin."

"I agree, my darling husband, about Jim-Niacin's abilities, if humans would just give him a chance he would save most of the lower extremities that are being lost because of Mr. Diabetes Disease."

The Captain got up from his recliner, walked over to Jan and gave her a warm tender kiss on her waiting luscious lips and said, "I'm off to bed, dear, I'll wait up for you."
"I won't be long, dear," said Jan.

        Things had been rather calm in Health-land Kingdom for the last few months VC, VE, and John-pyridoxine all were very busy taking care of the town's population. About the only thing going on was the mayoral election coming up very soon.

They all thought the town hall meeting did a lot of good for the community. They felt it educated the citizens that there was a lot they could do for themselves concerning their health care.

That means that one will not have   to jump on the super MD highway for the slightest little pin prick or minor inconvenience. Sure, there is only so much we vitamins, minerals, herbs, etc. can do to promote health, we don't try to be everything to everybody.
After the town hall meeting Mr.

Disease was steaming mad. He was even thinking of calling a meeting of all the different diseases. The nerve of those vitamins, minerals, humans, herbs and other nutrients trying to get together and put him and his friends out of business.

They want to try to put his most successful friends like cancer, diabetes, heart disease, and AIDS out of business. He was not having it; that was not going to be tolerated. Mr. Disease started planning.

He would try to attack their left flank by bringing back some of his old friends like the Black Plague, Tuberculosis, and West Nile, next he would try to rush their right flank with AIDS to try to split their force, then he would try to rout them up the middle with lots of Cancer and Heart Disease.

I will take no prisoners. Who do they think this is, this is Mr. Disease and I don't play, I even quit school because they had recess. It is on. How dare they have this town hall meeting to try and get rid of me and my friends.

After a long hot summer the day of the mayoral election had finally arrived and it looked like it was going to be a big turn out. At seven o'clock p.m. Captain Fredrico, Jan, Bob, and Melinda had comfortable seats at election headquarters. All of the election precincts closed at seven o'clock p.m. sharp.

The captain and his family started watching the tally on the big electronic board as the precincts came in. Captain Fredrico jumped out to an early four point lead and was able to maintain the lead throughout the night as the precincts came in. Then, finally the election supervisor announced, "Citizens of Health-land Kingdom the mayor elect is Orry Fredrico." Within seconds several microphones were thrust in Captain Fredrico's face.

A reporter was almost yelling, "Captain Fredrico, how does it feel being the mayor elect of Health-land Kingdom."

"First, I would like to thank my family and all of the volunteers that worked so hard on my behalf to make this   happen. Next, I would like to thank all of the citizens of Health-land Kingdom who had the faith and trust in me and backed it up by turning out to vote for me.

"Also, I would like to inform those that did not vote for me that I will be mayor of all the citizens of Health-land Kingdom. Finally, I would like to thank my opponent for a good clean hard fought campaign. Thanks again everyone. Good night."

Chapter 7

    About one month after Captain Fredrico had been sworn in as mayor of Health-land Kingdom, he announced that the first Saturday in March would be recognized by the town as Jim-Niacin's day.

On the morning of the first Saturday in March Mayor Fredrico stood at the podium at Healthy living park before a very large crowd.

"Citizens of Health-land Kingdom, today as your mayor I am proclaiming today as Jim-Niacin's day. We have on hand plenty of free food, drinks, and entertainment. To kick off this festive day, I'm going to deliver this short speech about the vitamin citizen we are celebrating today.

"Citizens of Health-land, Jim-Niacin is sort of an enigma. Many here had never heard of him, and of those that had, many of them fear and hate him. Still there is a great many that love this vitamin to death.

"I myself am one of those that dearly love Jim-Niacin and the good work he does. I am not telling you what I heard about Jim-Niacin, I'm telling you what I've personally experienced with my dealing with Jim-Niacin. I'm giving it to you first hand, straight from the horse's mouth.

"As I've told my wife and many others, I don't care what anyone says, to me Jim-Niacin is a miracle vitamin. This small, quiet, lowly member of the powerful B vitamin family is a Godsend as far as I'm concerned. As a proud virile human male I think of the many, many years that I suffered with extremely dry skin.

"For years I tried everything to get relief from this annoying dry skin condition. Even at the cure all metropolis they just prescribed an extremely expensive body cream that did little better than cheap over-the-counter lotions.

"Bathing and warm water had become the enemy. Washing only arm pits and the private area was becoming the norm, and I just hated my predicament. To me cleanliness is next to Godliness.

"Sure, I had heard of Jim-Niacin,

but it was mainly bad stuff, I never knew about his real power until I attended the town hall meeting. Over the years the dry skin problem was getting worse. Some type of fungus had invaded my toe nails and my skin was losing its luster in a few locations.

"The battle for healthy skin was a battle I knew I was losing , but no one could help me and I didn't know what to do. All of my life I've never been a quitter, I knew there was an answer, the problem was finding it, so I just kept on searching and searching.

"I was at my wits end, nothing or no one seemed able to help me find relief from my extremely dry skin condition. Then, at the final hour when all seemed lost and there was no hope left, Jim-Niacin came riding in on a big white horse at the town hall meeting.

"At the town hall meeting Jim-Niacin gave out his unclogging dose of 250 mg. twice a day after a meal.

The first thing is I must warn you that taking Jim-Niacin's unclogging dose is no cake walk or stroll through the park. That is the reason many who have tried taking Jim's doses don't like him and is afraid of him.

"When Jim goes to work unclogging those capillaries and small blood vessels it is not pleasant by any means. This flushing process varies in intensity, sometimes it may be mild, then at other times your skin may feel like it is literally on fire.

"This flushing process may last anywhere from five to thirty minutes, but seldom lasts more than thirty minutes. I have no evidence to support this, but I believe diabetes itself is caused by a deficiency in niacin, chromium, and a few other nutrients.

"Citizens of Health-land I could go on and on praising Jim-Niacin because in the past he truly has been an unsung hero. I will add this and come to a close. Don't ever go over his maximum 500 mg. daily dose or it could cause liver damage.

"In closing, I will assure you that his unclogging dose got rid of my dandruff, dry skin, toe nail fungus, etc. Stand up Jim-Niacin and say a few words," concluded Captain Fredrico.

As Jim-Niacin arrived at the podium he stood tall and proud. The audience went wild with applause, then chanted, "We love you Jim, we love you Jim, we love you "Thank you, thank you, thank you," said Jim-Niacin, "and may God bless this great town and keep it healthy always."

THE END

Chapter 8

     Freddie L. Sirmans was born in Stockton, Georgia on December 22,

1942.   In 1956 he moved with his
family to 717 East Cunning Street,
Valdosta, Georgia at the age of
Fourteen.

He finished Pinevale High
School in Valdosta in 1961. He
Turned down a basketball scholarship
To attend Fort Valley State College in
Georgia upon graduation.

In late 1962 Mr. Sirmans enlisted
In the U.S. Air Force where he
Became a fire and crash rescue man
And fire fighter.

After four years in the U.S. Air
Force Mr. Sirmans returned to
Valdosta in 1966. In 1969 he married
Carolyn Laverne Cunningham. That
Union ended in a divorce in 1980.

He has operated several small
Businesses and help raise four kids,
Felicia Regina Sirmans, Freddie Lee
Sirmans Jr., Hoover Charles
Sirmans and Erica Laverne Sirmans.

He is dedicating this book to his

Grand kids, Zaporia Monique Bass, Hoover Charles Sirmans II, Felicia Yvette Sirmans, Freddie Lee Sirmans III, Ayana Nicole Sirmans Fellows, Amari Jordan Sirmans, Tommy Elijah Sirmans, Cameron Alexander Sirmans, and Julia Sirmans.

The author believes strongly in The power of positive thinking. This Means you take a positive quote and Repeat it to yourself at least 50 or More times a day. The following are Some of the most powerful positive Quotes the author has used to survive Over the years.

1. "I can face and do all things Through God who strengthens me," (Paraphrased).

2. "I can face and forgive anything or Anybody," (optional) through God who Strengthens me.

3. I can wish all people goodwill no matter it its not returned.

4. I can face all threats and Imaginations.

5. "I can love and forgive all of my

looks And actions," (optional) through
God Who strengthens me?

Utilizing these positive thinking
Quotes will guarantee success to
Anyone who sticks with them.
It may take six months or more,
But sooner or later out of nowhere the
Inner faith and goodwill will be there.

BEWARE:
You can use only one quote at a time
During a six months period for the
Process to be effective.

MISCELLANEOUS
READING

WITH THANKSGIVING LET YOUR
REQUESTS BE KNOWN INTO GOD.
        (PARAPHRASED) PHIL. 4:6

 I CAN DO ALL THINGS THROUGH GOD
WHO STRENGTHENS ME.

(PARAPHRASED) PHIL. 4:13

THE LATTER WHEN REPEATED 50
OR MORE TIME A DAY WILL
GUARANTEE SELF CONFIDENCE
AND SUCCESS.

GUN SAFETY   RULES

1.   Never forget, that saying I'm sorry
and feeling sorry will not bring back a
life.

2.   To all kids, if you find a gun,
Never touch it or play with it, don't
Wait, go! Go! Go find an adult or call
an adult. Don't listen to little Johnny or
Susie, go! Go! Go!

II   GUN HANDLING SAFETY

1.   The gun safety should be on at all
times until ready to fire.

2.   A gun should be treated as if it is
loaded at all times, even when you

know it is not, meaning you should never point it toward anyone or snap the trigger unless the gun is pointed up or down.

3.   A gun must never be transported while loaded. when arriving at the hunting site, then load your gun. Again before leaving the hunting site unload you gun.

4.   During hunting your gun must always be carried pointed up or down.

5.   Never fire on level while hunting because a bullet travels a mile or more and could hit someone.

6.   In case of misfire keep your gun pointed in a safe direction, then count to ten before ejecting cartridge.

7.   Learning how to aim your gun: Most front sights are round shaped and the rear sights are U shaped, so when looking through your sight the round sight should be kept in the center of the U.

8.   When firing, the trigger should always be squeezed slowly, never a sudden pull or jerk.

9.   When shooting at a target the Front round dot sight must be kept in the center of the U sighting and should always be seen very clearly and your target seen only as a blur.

10. If the target you are shooting at is very clear, then you are going to miss because your target should always be blurred and only the dot in your sighting seen very clearly. Never at anytime get dirt into the barrel of your gun or any other part because it may blow it apart.
   Take care of your gun by cleaning and oiling it regular.

     I WILL LIFT UP MINE EYES UNTO THE HILLS, FROM WHENCE COMETH MY HELP. MY HELP COMETH FROM THE LORD, WHICH MADE HEAVEN AND EARTH. HE WILL NOT

SUFFER THY FOOT TO BE MOVED: HE THAT KEEPETH THEE WILL NOT SLUMBER. BEHOLD, HE THAT KEEPETH ISRAEL SHALL NEITHER SLUMBER NOR SLEEP. THE LORD IS THY KEEPER: THE LORD IS THY SHADE UPON THY RIGHT HAND. THE SUN SHALL NOT SMITE THEE BY DAY, OR THE MOON BY NIGHT. THE LORD SHALL PRESERVE THEE FROM ALL EVIL: HE SHALL PRESERVE THY SOUL. THE LORD SHALL PRESERVE THY GOING OUT AND THY COMING IN FROM THIS TIME FORTH, AND EVEN FOR EVERMORE.

121ST. PSALM

THE LORD IS MYSHEPHERD: I SHALL NOT WANT. HE MAKETH ME TO LIE DOWN IN GREEN PASTURES: HE LEADETH ME BESIDE THE STILL WATERS. HE RESTORETH MY SOUL: HE LEADETH ME IN THE PATHS OF RIGHTEOUSNESS FOR HIS NAME'S SAKE. YEA, THOUGH I WALK THROUGH THE VALLEY OF THE

SHADOW OF DEATH. I WILL FEAR NO
EVIL: FOR THOU ART WITH ME; THY
ROD AND THY STAFF THEY COMFORT
ME. THOU PREPAREST A TABLE
BEFORE ME IN THE PRESENCE OF
MINE ENEMIES: THOU ANOINTEST MY
HEAD WITH OIL; MY CUP
RUNNETH OVER. SURELY
GOODNESS AND MERCY SHALL
FOLLOW ME ALL THE DAYS OF MY
LIFE: AND I WILL DWELL IN THE
HOUSE OF THE LORD FOREVER.
                    23RD. PSALM

MAKE A JOYFUL NOISE UNTO THE
LORD, ALL YE LANDS. SERVE THE
LORD WITH GLADNESS: COME
BEFORE HIS PRESENCE WITH
SINGING. KNOW YE THAT THE LORD
HE IS GOD: IT IS HE THAT HATH
MADE US, AND NOT WE OURSELVES;
WE ARE HIS PEOPLE, AND THE SHEEP
OF HIS PASTURE. ENTER INTO HIS
GATES WITH THANKSGIVING, AND
INTO HIS COURTS WITH PRAISE: BE
THANKFUL INTO HIM, AND BLESS HIS

NAME. FOR THE LORD IS GOOD; HIS
MERCY IS EVERLASTING; AND HIS
TRUTH ENDURETH TO ALL
GENERATIONS.

100TH. PSALM

I CAN DO ALL THINGS THROUGH GOD
WHO STRENGTHENS ME.

(PARAPHRASED)
PHILIPPIANS 4.13

OH, I HAVE SLIPPED THE SURLY
BONDS OF EARTH AND DANCED
THE SKIES ON LAUGHTER-
SILVERED WINGS; SUNWARD I'VE
CLIMBED, AND JOINED THE TUMBLING
MIRTH OF SUN-SPLIT CLOUDS, AND
DONE A HUNDRED THINGS
YOU HAVE NOT DREAMED OF,
WHEELED AND SOURED AND
HIGH IN THE SUN LIT SILENCE.
HOV'RING THERE, I'VE CHASED
THE SHOUTING WIND ALONG,

AND FLUNG MY EAGER CRAFT
THROUGH FOOTLESS HALLS OF
AIR. UP, UP THE LONG,
DELIRIOUS, BURNING BLUE
I'VE TOPPED THE WINDSWEPT
HEIGHTS WITH EASY GRACE
WHERE NEVER LARK, OR EVEN
EAGLE FLEW.AND, WHILE WITH
SILENT, LIFTING MIND I'VE TROD THE
HIGH UNTRESPASSED SANCTITY OF
SPACE, PUT OUT MY HAND, AND
TOUCHED THE FACE OF GOD.

HIGHFLIGHT
BY JOHN GILLESPIE MAGEE, JR.

SHOULD | AULD AC-QUAINTANCE | BE
FOR-GOT, AND | NEV-ER BROUGHT
TO | MIND?   SHOULD | AULD   AC-
QUAIN-TANCE | BE   FOR-GOT, AND- |
DAYS OF AULD LANG | SYNE   FOR
| AULD-----LANG----|SYNE,   MY
DEAR,   FOR | AULD----LANG---- |
SYNE   WE'LL | TAK' A   CUP   O'
| KIND-NESS YET   FOR- | AULD----
LANG----| SYNE   AULD----LANG----
SYNE

FAMOUS NEW YEAR EVE SONG

OUR FATHER, WHICH ART IN HEAVEN, HALLOWED BE THY NAME. THY KINGDOM COMES. THY WILL BE DONE ON EARTH, AS IT IS IN HEAVEN. GIVE US THIS DAY OUR DAILY BREAD, AND FORGIVE US OUR DEBTS, AS WE FORGIVE OUR DEBTORS. AND LEAD US NOT INTO TEMPTATION, BUT DELIVER US FROM EVIL; FOR THINE IS THE KINGDOM, AND THE POWER, AND THE GLORY, FOREVER.   AMEN.

THE LORD'S PRAYER

WE THE PEOPLE OF THE UNITED STATES, IN ORDER TO FORM A MORE PERFECT UNION, ESTABLISH JUSTICE,

INSURE DOMESTIC TRANQUILLITY, PROVIDE FOR THE COMMON DEFENSE, PROMOTE THE GENERAL WELFARE, AND SECURE THE BLESSINGS OF LIBERTY TO OURSELVES AND OUR POSTERITY, DO ORDAIN AND ESTABLISH THIS CONSTITUTION FOR THE UNITED STATES OF AMERICA.

PREAMBLE TO THE CONSTITUTION FOR THE UNITED STATES OF AMERICA

I PLEDGE ALLEGIANCE TO THE FLAG OF THE UNITED STATES OF AMERICA AND TO THE REPUBLIC FOR WHICH IT STANDS: ONE NATION UNDER GOD, INDIVISIBLE, WITH LIBERTY AND JUSTICE FOR ALL.

THE PLEDGE WAS FIRST USED ON OCT. 12, 1892, DURING COLUMBUS DAY OBSERVANCES IN THE PUBLIC SCHOOLS. AMENDED: THE WORDS "FLAG OF THE UNITED STATES OF AMERICA"

INSTEAD OF "MY FLAG" OFFICIALLY ON FLAG DAY, JUNE 14, 1924. AGAIN AMENDED IN 1954 BY THE ADDITION OF THE WORDS "UNDER GOD."

CONGRESS SHALL MAKE NO LAW RESPECTING AN ESTABLISHMENT OF RELIGION, OR PROHIBITING THE FREE EXERCISE THEREOF; OR ABRIDGING THE FREEDOM OF SPEECH, OR OF THE PRESS, OR THE RIGHT OF THE PEOPLE PEACEABLY TO ASSEMBLE, AND TO PETITION THE GOVERNMENT FOR A REDRESS OF GRIEVANCES.

AMENDMENT I TO THE CONSTITUTION OF THE UNITED STATES OF AMERICA. AMENDMENTS I-X IS KNOWN AS THE BILL OF RIGHTS.

THE POWERS NOT DELEGATED

TO THE UNITED STATES BY THE CONSTITUTION, NOR PROHIBITED BY IT TO THE STATES, ARE RESERVED TO THE STATES RESPECTIVELY, OR TO THE PEOPLE.

AMENDMENT X TO THE CONSTITUTION OF THE UNITED STATES OF AMERICA.

NEITHER SLAVERY NOR INVOLUNTARY SERVITUDE, EXCEPT AS A PUNISHMENT FOR CRIME WHEREOF THE PARTY SHALL HAVE BEEN DULY CONVICTED, SHALL EXIST WITHIN THE UNITED STATES, OR ANY PLACE SUBJECT TO THEIR JURISDICTION.

AMENDMENT XIII TO THE CONSTITUTION OF THE UNITED STATES OF AMERICA.
RATIFIED DECEMBER 6, 1865.

GOD HELPS THOSE WHO FIRST
HELP THEM.

TO TRY AND KEEP TRYING IS THE
GREATEST OF ALL VIRTUES.
                    Author ?

NOTHING CAN TAKE THE PLACE OF
PERSISTENCE. INTELLIGENCE AND
ABILITY WILL NOT; TALENT AND
SKILL WILL NOT; NOTHING IS MORE
COMMON THAN UNSUCCESSFUL
PEOPLE WITH INTELLIGENCE AND
ABILITY; THE WORLD IS FULL OF
EDUCATED FAILURES. PERSISTENCE
AND DETERMINATION ALONE WILL
GUARANTEE SUCCESS.
                    Author ?

"THE SONG"

O SAY CAN YOU SEE,
BY THE DAWN'S EARLY LIGHT,WHAT
SO PROUDLY WE HAIL'D AT THE
TWILIGHT'S LAST GLEAMING,WHOSE
BROAD STRIPES AND BRIGHT
STARS THROUGH THE PERILOUS
FIGHT O' ER THE RAMPARTS WE
WATCHED, WERE SO GALLANTLY
STREAMING? AND THE ROCKET'S RED
GLARE, THE BOMBS BURSTING IN
AIR,GAVE PROOF THROUGH THE
NIGHT THAT OUR FLAG WAS STILL
THERE, O SAY DOES THAT STAR-
SPANGLED BANNER YET WAVE
O' ER THE LAND OF THE FREE
AND THE HOME OF THE BRAVE?

SMARTER STUDENTS MEANS BETTER STUDENTS

MANY PUBLIC LEADERS ARE
TRYING VERY HARD TO FIGURE
OUT HOW TO IMPROVE OUR

PUBLIC SCHOOLS. WELL, THE ANSWER IS VERY SIMPLE. IN ORDER TO HAVE BETTER SCHOOLS, YOU FIRST MUST HAVE SMARTER STUDENTS. ON THE SURFACE THAT SOUNDS LIKE A QUIP ANSWER, BUT SINCE THE STRONG FAMILY INFLUENCE IS ON THE DECLINE, THERE DOESN'T SEEM TO BE THAT STRONG DISCIPLINE THAT IS NEEDED TO FORCE MANY OF TODAY'S KIDS TO READ AND STUDY HARD LIKE IN PAST YEARS.   IN MANY FAMILIES A CYCLE OF IGNORANCE HAS BUILT UP AND I FEEL NOTHING YOU DO IS GOING TO WORK UNLESS THAT CYCLE IS BROKEN. I FEEL THE ONLY THING THAT WILL BREAK GENERATIONS OF IGNORANCE IS TO READ, READ, READ, AND KEEP READING. I FEEL EVERY SCHOOL AND PUBLIC LIBRARY IN THE COUNTRY OUGHT TO HAVE SOME KIND OF PROGRAM TO REWARD KIDS FOR READING BOOKS. IT DOESN'T HAVE TO BE MUCH MAYBE A FEW DOLLARS OR SOME KIND OF REWARD WOULD MEAN

A LOT TO A POOR KID AND WOULD
TEACH HIM THAT WHAT HE GETS OUT
OF LIFE, DEPENDS ON HIS OWN
ACTIONS. REWARDING READERS
WOULD BE ESPECIALLY HELPFUL TO
INNER CITY YOUTHS AND IS
PROBABLE THE ONLY THING
THAT WILL FREE ON A LARGE
SCALE, MANY GENERATIONS OF
MYTHS AND NEGATIVE THINKING.

FREDDIE L. SIRMANS, SR.
MAY 3, 1998 LETTER TO THE
EDITOR

"IT IS NOT THE CRITIC THAT
COUNTS; NOT THE MAN WHO
POINTS OUT HOW THE STRONG
MAN STUMBLES, OR WHERE THE
DOER OF DEEDS COULD HAVE DONE
THEM BETTER. THE CREDIT BELONGS
TO THE MAN WHO IS ACTUALLY IN
THE ARENA, WHOSE FACE IS MARRED
BY DUST AND SWEAT AND BLOOD;
WHO STRIVES VALIANTLY; WHO ERRS,
AND COMES UP SHORT AGAIN AND

AGAIN, BECAUSE THERE IS NO EFFORT WITHOUT ERROR AND SHORTCOMING; BUT WHO DOES ACTUALLY STRIVE TO
DO THE DEEDS; WHO KNOWS THE GREAT ENTHUSIASMS, THE GREAT DEVOTIONS; WHO SPENDS HIMSELF IN WORTHY CAUSE; WHO AT BEST KNOWS IN THE END THE TRIUMPH OF HIGH ACHIEVEMENT, AND WHO AT WORSE, IF HE FAILS, AT LEAST FAILS WHILE DARING GREATLY, SO THAT HIS PLACE SHALL NEVER BE WITH THOSE COLD AND TIMID SOULS WHO KNOW NEITHER VICTORY NOR DEFEAT."
                    Author ?

A 3 PRONG WEIGHT LOSING GAMBIT

I. **THE DIET ASPECT**

It helps to have a staple food. Many people use rice, potatoes, bread, or pasta as a staple, and serve one or the other almost every meal. These foods are all starches, which is fine,

but the portions should be kept small. It's far better to change to one or a combination of the following foods to use as a staple, such as green beans, mushrooms, broccoli, cauliflower, or any type of leafy vegetable, then the portions can be as large as you like. All fats should be kept to a minimum.
It's best to use oils high in Omega-3 fatty acids such as canola oil, or olive oil. A lot of the vital nutrients are missing from highly processed food. Also, there is wide use of antibiotics in the meat raising process, plus the use of all kinds of pesticides and herbicides in growing our food. With this going on our immune system need all of the help it can get through vitamins and mineral supplements.
A rule of thumb for the hard to lose weight fighters should be to limit the following "big 5" foods, rice, potatoes, bread, pasta, and artificial sweets. If that rule is obeyed, then it's true one can eat all he wants and still lose weight. Some starch is needed to prevent indigestion,

preferable a small amount of stone grounded wheat breads each meal.
PROSTATE DISEASE
AND IMPOTENCY PROTECTION
FOR MEN: Daily supplements, 50 mg of zinc, 1000 mg of pumpkin seed oil, 1 capsules of 160mg of saw palmetto extract twice a day, 1000i.u. of vitamin E, and 250 mg of niacin. When first taking niacin the unclogging of the capillaries sometime gives one's skin a normal hot flushing feeling for a few minutes. Just remember that is
normal when taking niacin.
ANOTHER GREAT BENEFIT FOR THOSE OVER WEIGHT TO ELIMINATE THE BIG 5 FOODS IS: If one then takes a chromium tablet at each meal it should control high blood sugar with most people.

II. **THE PHYSICAL ASPECT**
Anyone wanting to lose weight needs to first maintain a healthy body, and that can't be done without some type of exercise. It's a fact that one in good physical

condition has as much as ten times a better chance of surviving a heart attack, stroke, or any kind of ailment than someone not in shape. Almost everyone can take a brisk walk for 25 minutes or more at least 3 times a week.
There is no excuse, some type of exercise such as walking, weight lifting, etc. must be done to maintain a healthy body. To keep ones fuel burning (metabolism) rate at its maximum one needs to eat 3 regular meals and a snack or two, plus some exercise each day. When one misses a meal the body automatically starts conserving energy and will burn very few calories.

III. **THE MENTAL ASPECT**
It's a fact that ninety five percent of the people that lose weight have regained it all back and more after five years. I believe that is because the mental aspect is almost always ignored. To deal with the mental aspect, I've thought up a

positive thinking quote that must be repeated to oneself a minimum of 50 times each day.

Never quit saying the quote because it may take six months or longer to fully kick in. You can't will a positive thought, the result comes through the repeating process itself. The process can be speeded up by increasing the number of times repeated each day. Just repeat this quote "A little bit of food is all I want," Don't quit! Give it time! It works! Upon completion most fast eaters will always want more, but if they can just hold off for 10 minutes that desire should be gone.

THE END

Novel:
A SECOND CHANCE TO LIVE II
CHAPTER 1

Rufus Thomas was relaxed and happy

on this Friday afternoon as he was taking down the   steam-table out front in the dining room, when all of a sudden he heard shots and glass breaking. Then it occurred to him like being awaken out of a dream, that someone was shooting into the restaurant. Without a second of delay, he instinctively fell to the floor.

As he lay on the floor his mind raced back to an incident that had happened in his parking lot about a week ago. Within the last two weeks, a group of young teenagers had started using his parking lot to make drug deals. So last week, he decided to put a stop to it.

He put his 9mm(9 millimeter semi-automatic hand gun) in his pocket and walked out to the parking lot keeping his hand in his pocket on his gun. "Hey you kids, don't y'all know this is private property?" said Rufus in a strong firm voice. One of the kids, who looked to be around 15 or 16 replied, "we have a right to be here."

"Not on my property you don't. I'm telling you to get off my property right now before I call the cops."

"And if we don't?"

"That's your choice."

After swearing and grumbling, they slowly moved off down the street. After a couple of days Rufus decided to put the incident out of his mind.

A voice yelling, "Mr. Thomas, Mr. Thomas are you all right?" brought him back to the present and to his feet. It was Zaporia Monique one of the two waitresses that worked for him. "Mr. Thomas; what happen? are you all right?"

"I think so Zaporia, someone was shooting through the windows. I believe those kids I ran off the property about a week ago had something to do with this."

Erica the other waitress who worked at the restaurant had come out of the kitchen to see what all of the commotion was about. "It's okay, Erica Laverne you and Zaporia go ahead and finish cleaning up, I'm going to call the police."

CHAPTER 2

Bruce Allen was born in Buieville, GA., he learned early growing up in the Jimmy Carroll housing projects that you had to watch your back and fight to survive. Bruce loved his mother with all his heart but had only contempt for a father he had never met who deserted his mother before he was born.

His mother tried her best to make him go to school, but he had become more interested in making money. He had learned that money meant power, the ability to get pretty women, and the nice things in life. The youth gang in the Jimmy Carroll housing projects was called The Young Vipers. The Young Vipers' ages ranged from twelve to sixteen.

Bruce joined The Young Vipers as soon as he became eligible. By the time Bruce turned age fifteen, he was the undisputed leader of The Young Vipers. No one becomes a leader of the gang without being brutal, cunning, and savage. Some things Bruce Allen could forgive a person for, but disrespecting him was the unforgivable sin, and whoever crossed that boundary had to pay.

Growing up in the Jimmy Carroll housing projects, Bruce was no stranger to the drug business. As long as he could remember, the most successful people he knew were drug dealers. They had money, pretty women, and new cars. What else could one want? That was everything. At a very young age Bruce started in the drug business at the very bottom.

For a few dollars he would work as a lookout for the dealers and warn them if the cops were approaching. Now, he had graduated to doing a little dealing himself. Last Friday down on Mary Alice Ave., Bruce was about to close his biggest drug deal yet, when this old stooge had to come out and mess everything up. It is a perfect location for dealing drugs.

It is located off to the side where you can see who is approaching from a great distance. This is a free country, he thought. Who does that old stooge think he is going around disrespecting people?

A few days after the incident, Bruce and a

few of The Young Vipers were hanging out at Regina's Cafe Bruce, still fuming about being disrespected Bruce said to his second in command, "You know, Boom Boom, that parking lot down on Mary Alice Ave. is the best drug dealing location I know of.

"You're right Bruce," replied Boom Boom, "we could have that parking lot all to ourselves if nobody was in that building.   I think if somebody stole a car, drove by, and shot up the place that would teach that old stooge a lesson."

"Boom Boom, I Believe you're right," said Bruce.

CHAPTER 3

At Buieville Police Department on Friday afternoon,
Lieutenant Marvin Elder was anticipating a relaxed weekend with his family. Maybe we'll take the boat out on the lake for a few hours he thought. Lt. Elder came from a long line of lawmen; his granddad was a deputy sheriff and two of his uncles were policemen. But his father didn't want any part of law enforcement. His father became a fire fighter.

After over eighteen years on the Buieville Police Department Lt. Elder was nearing retirement. He started off as a foot patrolman in and around the Jimmy Carroll housing projects, which is one of the roughest neighborhoods in the city. Over the years, he served in the Traffic Division, Detective Division, Internal Affairs Division, and NARC. Division. Then about a year ago, they picked him to head up the new Youth Gang Division.

Lt. Elder was in the process of finishing up his daily reports, when his secretary Carolyn Laverne yelled, "Lt., pick up line two."

"This is Lt. Marvin Elder may I help you?"

"Lt. Elder this is Rufus Thomas, I operate The Harlem Garden Restaurant at 1401 S. Mary Alice Ave. We just had a drive by shooting down here."

"Was anybody hurt? "asked Lt. Elder.

"Fortunately not, I was the only one out front in the dining area; luckily my two waitresses were back in the kitchen. Also, I hit the deck after the first blast."

"Did you see the car that did the shooting?"

"Before I hit the deck I caught a glimpse of gray, but I couldn't tell what make or model it was." "

"Do you know how many shots were fired?"

"I can't be for sure. Maybe three or four shots, everything happened so fast I just can't be for sure."

"Mr. Thomas have you had any dissatisfied customers or disputes with anyone recently."

"Yes, as a matter of fact I believe I know who is behind this whole thing. It began about two weeks ago when some teenagers started what looked to me like drug dealing in my parking lot."

"Did you call the police?"

"Maybe I should have. But you know how it is, drugs are so bad. You know they are going to do them; you just hope they do them somewhere else. But last Friday afternoon I got fed up and went out there and told them to get off my property, or I would call the cops."

"Mr. Thomas, I need to warn you. You are definitely risking your life confronting these gangs. They are young, but don't let that fool you; these kids are gang members and they will not hesitate to hurt you. Mr. Thomas, it will take me about thirty minutes to get down there to investigate the scene and ask you a few more questions."

"Maybe I can track down this gang who has started using your parking lot. But Mr. Thomas, I suggest you take precaution, because this drive by shooting is probably the first attack in a war on you and your property."

While pulling into the parking lot at the Harlem Garden Restaurant, Lt. Elder's professional trained eye alertly surveyed the parking lot and surrounding area.

He quickly saw why someone dealing drugs would like this location. The parking lot was located on the side of the building with just enough shrubbery to conceal a small group of people. It was isolated enough to allow early warning when someone was approaching. The restaurant was not very large, it probably had a seating capacity of around fifty people.   The building and landscape were clean and well kept.

Pushing through the front door, he quickly noticed the liberal use of wood grain and honey colored paneling. He sensed that he would be dealing with a very conservative individual. The color scheme was pine green, navy blue, with a few spots of burgundy. The place seemed almost regal. It definitely was no cheap greasy spoon.

He noticed a man behind the serving line. "Hello sir, I'm Lt. Elder from Buieville P.D.."

"Hello, Lt. I'm Rufus Thomas the owner of this restaurant."
Lt. Elder walked to the back wall opposite the two bullet shattered front windows. Reaching into his pocket he pulled out a small leathermen's tool, then he proceeded to dig out what looked like a 9mm slug.

He next found three other bullet holes. "Mr. Thomas, your estimation of the number of shots seems to be right," said Lt. Elder. "In all I counted four bullet holes. Mr. Thomas, I would like for you to tell me everything you can think of about the kids you ran off your property last week. Did you notice anything unusual or out of the ordinary? Did you notice any scars, any limps, speech impediment, or anything that may help to identify this gang?"

There are over fifty gangs in this city, it is almost like finding a needle in a hay stack. "I'm sorry Lt., they just seem like ordinary kids," said Mr. Thomas.

"Here is my card, Mr. Thomas, please give me a call if you think of anything later that might help me find this gang. Also, give me a call if you see anything that's out of the ordinary, like the same car going past your restaurant more than normal."

"I certainly will, thank you Lt," said Mr. Thomas.

CHAPTER 4

Janet Thomas loved her work as a nurse at Betty Gertrude
Memorial Hospital. Ever since she was a little girl she had wanted to help and care for people. On Fridays Janet loved to have dinner out or have some friends over. But it's been a while since she shared a quiet dinner at home alone with her husband Rufus.

Janet eased her brand new, willow green and burgundy colored vinyl top Towncar into traffic. She was accustomed to the thirty minute drive to their ranch style home on Debra Marie
Drive in Woodgate Heights. As the town car begin to cruise, Janet thought back to when she was twenty-years old. Then Janet Brown,

she attended Walter Bernard Community College in San Diego. She remembered, through her best friend Minnie Martin, she was introduced to a young Navy Petty Officer named Rufus Thomas.

At first he seemed too serious and no nonsensical for her taste, but slowly she realized it was a facade to cover up his real shyness. Underneath he had a genuine dry wit sense of humor. As Debra Marie Drive came into view, it brought Janet back to the present.

She checked her watch as she slowed the Towncar and turned right onto Debra Marie Dr. The time was five P.M. She was expecting her husband Rufus to arrive home around five thirty.

Leroy Jackson and Rufus Thomas had been friends ever since their high school days. Not a week went by that they didn't go fishing, bowling, play a game of chess, or do something together. Leroy's wife Patricia hated Rufus' political views. Leroy's political views tended to be moderate, but his wife Pat was a true bleeding heart liberal.

Pat was always telling him, "For the life of me Leroy I don't see why you like to hang around with that damn Rufus Thomas. I believe he is some kind of extremist rightwing nut or something.

Always blaming everything on big government and the welfare state. How the hell does he think poor people and the homeless are going to survive without welfare and food stamps. I can't pay my bills as it is. I'm down to my last dollar. I sure hope they hurry up and call my number on the lottery."

Leroy enjoyed their friendship. Most of what Rufus said went in one ear and out the other. But Rufus was right about welfare and the social programs destroying the family and the extended family unit in this country.

Before pushing the key pad buttons to arm the security system and lock the front door, Rufus decided he best take Lt. Elder's advice on being cautious. He didn't always carry his handgun on him, but until this gang was caught, he planned on being prepared to defend himself at all times. He put his 9mm in his pocket and locked up.

As he merged his Silverado into traffic heading home, he thought every American should thank God they lived in a country with the freedom to bear arms, it is the rare exception; not the rule. Liberals are spouting the big lie when they say it would be safer with no guns. The real threat to our freedom and safety is not the criminal with a gun, he is only doing what he is allowed to do.

The real threat to our freedom and

safety is the shallow minded liberals who allow creeping socialism to prevail. The main reason the founding fathers enacted the second amendment was not for hunting and personal protection, but as a last resort to save individual freedom from an all powerful government out of control.   The fact is, there is no way we could have and continue to keep the freedoms we take for granted in this country without the freedom to possess arms. It was almost six p.m. when Rufus eased his Silverado into his carport.

After quietly letting himself in the carport door, he heard the pleasant voice of his wife saying, "Hello dear."

"Hello," said Rufus walking over to the counter near the

" said sink where she was making a salad. Rufus gave his wife a quick kiss on the lips. "Janet," said Rufus, "a bad thing happened at the restaurant today. We had a driveby shooting."

"Oh my God! Why would anybody want to do that?", she moaned.

"I can't be a hundred percent sure, but I believe some kids I ran off the property about a week ago had something to do with it. I told Lt. Elder from the Buieville Police Dept. about the kids I ran off the property, and he seems to think they belong to one of the youth gangs operating in the city. Lt. Elder also believes the gang has declared war on me and my property."

"Rufus, you know I have asked you in

the past to relocate your business out of that god forsaken area, you see how the surrounding neighborhoods have changed in the last few years."

"Gang or no gang, I am not going to let a group of kids run me off my property."

"But sweetheart, promise me you will at least consider relocating."

"Okay; I promise."

"Good, said Janet. "Now you go ahead and clean up; I'm preparing us a nice candle light dinner."

As the shower water sprayed over his body, Rufus let his mind drift back to when he was a young Navy Seaman stationed at San Diego. The Navy had trained him to be a cook, but on his off-duty time he decided to take English 101 at Walter Bernard Community College.

There he got to know a young lady in his English class named Minnie Martin. At a party, Minnie introduced him to Janet Brown. At first, he thought Janet was too much of the party type for him, but he soon realized she was one of the most selfless people he had ever known.

She loved her friends, but they would never take the place of a stable home life. They got engaged, and a year later they were married. The aroma of Janet's home cooking brought him back to the present. Once they sat down to the candle light dinner and the blessing was said, Rufus thought just how much he had to be thankful for.

He had a beautiful and charming wife, a lovely daughter, Freddy Mae, who had finished college and had a career of her own as a computer programmer, and most of all he still had his life, health, and strength. Hearing Janet say, "How do you like the food Rufus?" brought him out of his deep thoughts.

"Sweetheart, it tastes great, you know how I just love your down home cooking."

After the meal they moved to the sofa in the den. They sat side-by-side on the sofa with Janet leaning gently against his chest. As they listened to their favorite oldies, Rufus gently stroked and caressed Janet's neck and shoulder area. Every now and then he would kiss her gently.

As time passed, the kisses became regular, then, more regular and passionate, still, more regular and passionate, releasing his embrace, he gently lead her to the bedroom. Later as they lay in each others arms' totally spent, they told each other how much they loved each other. Relaxing in bed after making love, Rufus liked to express his political philosophy as long as Janet would stay awake.

Without a reply sometimes, he would talk for thirty minutes or more. "You know, Janet," said Rufus, "when I see young kids committing all of these crimes. Sure, you have to blame them primarily, but it goes much deeper. The real blame is the welfare state and the parents. All throughout history, the male carried out discipline in the home until within the last fifty years.

"Before fifty years ago this country never had a problem with family values or ill-raised youngsters. Then around fifty years ago, welfare and the social programs took over the role of provider and daddy, without enforcing discipline. The first thing the welfare and social provider did was demand that no man could live with his family if they received government aid. That order drove off the one that had maintained family values and discipline all throughout history.

"With welfare and social programs being the real provider, the on hand female became only a stand-in provider. Both of these new providers failed to carry out the first duty of being a provider. That primary duty was to maintain family discipline and values. With raising young men, some women can be tough and do a good job, but most can't or won't do the job.

Now, with the welfare and social program tentacles extending all throughout this society, true family discipline and family values in most cases are something from the past. That is the cause of our present state. Most of the kids in these gangs have never had any real discipline. These kids have never been conditioned to fear real punishment or consequences for improper behavior.

"The only way to bring back the strong

family and extended family system is for the government to wean itself out of the role of uncle sugar daddy. It's only since the big government sugar daddy booted the man, for the most part, out of the provider role that so many of our young men are being lost to drugs and violence.

"All that is necessary for us to solve our social problems is for the government to get out of people's lives as much as possible. Sure, there will be hardship and suffering, but it has to be a natural selection process, otherwise any do-good human tinkering is only going to compound the problem and make it worse.

"Another thing, is all of this hollering about jobs going overseas. What's missing here is the jobs are being driven overseas by big government, high health cost, high taxes, environmental laws, and other big government mandates.
" It's a matter of survival, no business can compete and survive unless it makes a profit. There must be something an ordinary citizen can do to make a difference." "Janet you know,
I think I'll try writing a book. Janet;" said Rufus a little louder.   zzzzz, zzzzz, zzzzz.

"Oh well, it was a good idea anyway," said Rufus as he turned over on his left side, his favorite sleeping position.

Tonight he was sure he would sleep like a baby.

CHAPTER 5

Bruce Allen was age sixteen, and his mother Miss Gracie Bell Allen thought he was in school everyday. Sure, Bruce would leave home every school day morning; but instead of going to school he would spend the day playing basketball and at his girl friend's LaTonya's house. LaTonya was on welfare, but you wouldn't know it because she lived in a nice home in a nice neighborhood.

LaTonya had just turned eighteen years old and had two kids. Bruce's favorite hangout was Regina's Cafe. Miss Felicia Regina, the lady that owns the cafe, would sometimes get her niece LaTonya to come down and help her out at the cafe. A little over a year ago, Bruce started trying to talk to LaTonya, but she wouldn't have anything to do him because she felt he was too young for her.

A few months later, some guy started giving LaTonya a hard time. After a while Bruce walked up to the guy and said in a low but strong, firm tone of voice, "Listen buddy, I'm going to ask you only one time to leave the lady alone." The guy just stared at Bruce for several seconds, then said, "So that's the way it is?"

"That's the way it is," replied Bruce. The guy said he didn't want any trouble and left.

About a week later, LaTonya invited Bruce over to her house. Now over a year later Bruce and LaTonya are still seeing each other. Bruce tells her he loves her and wants to buy her a car and some of the finer things in life. After spending most of the day with LaTonya, Bruce, Boom Boom, and a few other gang members were scheduled to meet that evening at Regina's Cafe for an important meeting.

Later that evening, Bruce told the gang members that he didn't want to kill the old stooge, he just wanted to drive him out of business and teach him a lesson. "Bruce, you must be getting a little soft. This guy is armed and dangerous," said Boom Boom.
Bruce thought that it may be only a matter of time before he would have to put Boom Boom in his place. "Okay," said Bruce, one last time, "Everyone is expected to have two cans of spray paint. We will arrive at the building in groups of three and leave in groups of three. The job shouldn't take over five minutes. The strike time is ten o'clock. Any questions? No questions? Then I'll see you guys tonight."

One advantage of being a long time cop is you have time to develop a lot of information sources. Monday morning Lt. Elder logged out to some of the roughest neighborhoods in the city. The first stop on his list was the Jimmy Carroll Housing Project.

Before leaving, he decided to give his secretary Carolyn Laverne some last minute instructions. "Carolyn, I want you to check with the record section and see if they have any reports of gray cars being stolen within the last week. If so, find out who found it and any information they have on it."

"Yes sir, I will take care of that right away."

"I'll be out of the office all morning, but I should be back around noon."

"I'll have my portable in case I have to be reached in an emergency."

"Yes sir." It had been quiet awhile since Lt. Elder had visited the Jimmy Carroll Housing Project.

His mind raced back to about thirty years ago when he was a young man. He remembered growing up in the Little Miami section not very far from the Jimmy Carroll Housing Project. Back then the projects were a very decent and respectable place to live. As a senior in high school, he use to play sand-lot football and date girls in the projects.

They had a fine community center and basketball courts. But like a lot of housing projects around the country, it has degenerated because of crime and drugs. To keep from completely losing it to crime and drugs the, Buieville Police Dept. located a precinct station there and started foot patrols. He was brought back to the present as the five story white brick buildings came into view.

Lt. Elder decided to park in front of the office but not because he had any intention of going inside. He was sure he still had a couple of long time contacts still around. Since it was about nine a.m., there was hardly anybody outside standing around. That suited him fine because a lot of people were suspicious of anyone talking to a cop for any reason.

Lt. Elder decided to try Littlejohn's apartment to see if he was home. After reaching Littlejohn's apartment, he pulled the screen door back and gave three loud, quick raps on the door. After a few seconds, he thought he heard a slight movement inside. Then after waiting several more seconds, he again gave three loud, quick raps. This time he was sure he definitely heard someone approaching the door. Then a voice barely audible from the inside said, "Who is it?"

"Lt. Elder."

"Who?"

"Lt. Elder," he said much louder.

"Just a minute." After what seemed like a full minute a, very small man cracked the door about six inches. "What can I do for you Lt.?" As Lt. Elder looked at Littlejohn he wondered what motivation, or lack of motivation causes people to throw away their life. Littlejohn stayed away from crack and the hard drugs, but as Lt. Elder peered at his face and eyes he could see that cheap wine and rot gut liquor had certainly taken its toll.

"Littlejohn, I would like to come in and talk to you for a couple of minutes," he said.

Littlejohn opened the door wide and stood aside. Lt. Elder strode inside a few feet, then pivoted around to face Littlejohn.

"Littlejohn, I want to know what the word on the street is if any, about a driveby shooting on the Harlem Garden Restaurant last week."

"The word is, it was one of the young gangs," said Littlejohn.

"Do you have any names?"

"No, that's all I've heard on it."

Lt. Elder reached into his pocket and pulled out a clip of bills and slid off a couple of twenties and told Littlejohn, "I Thomas want names."

"Give me a couple of days," said Littlejohn.

"Here is my card; give me a call the minute you get a name."

Leaving the Jimmy Carroll Housing Projects Lt. Elder then made a couple more contacts. The time was around noon so he decided to pick up some fried rice, sweet and sour pork, a couple of egg rolls and head on back to the office.

Rufus used to keep the Harlem Garden Restaurant open until 9 o'clock at night during the week and until 11 o'clock on Friday and Saturday nights. But about a year ago, he started closing around three thirty in the afternoon Monday through Thursday and nine p.m. on Friday and Saturdays because his older customers didn't like to come out at night due to crime.

Since the driveby shooting, Rufus made sure he was armed most of the time. He was constantly on the alert for any sign of trouble, but so far everything was quiet and normal around the Harlem Garden Restaurant. Rufus wanted to finish cleaning up and close on time this afternoon because Monday nights was his church league's bowling night.

Five members from their church made up their bowling team. The five members were Rufus Thomas, Leroy Jackson, Brenda Johnson, Danny Hebert, and Freddie Lee Jr. Rufus would usually pick up Leroy and they would meet the others at the bowling alley at 8 p.m. After Rufus finished watching the six o'clock news and Crossfire, he decided to go pick up Leroy and head to the bowling alley.

Pulling up at Leroy's house Rufus got out and rang the door bell. Rufus thought people who pulled up to a person's home and sit there blowing the horn were displaying laziness and ill manners. Why distract or wake up the whole neighborhood? Someone from inside the house said, "Who is it?"

"Rufus."

"I'm coming," said Leroy. By the time Rufus got back in the Silverado, Leroy was coming out the front door. "How is it going Rufus," said Leroy as he climbed in the passenger side of the Silverado.

"Doing pretty good; how about you?"

"I think I'll make it." Rufus backed the Silverado out and headed toward the bowling alley.

"Leroy," said Rufus, "do you think any one race is more intelligent than others?"

"I never thought much about it, but I don't think so," said Leroy.

"I don't think so either, but I do believe there might be a cultural factor that affects motivation.

" I believe motivation affect one's intelligence and achievement more than anything else in life, but it is almost always ignored. In every race there will be a smart high range and a dumb low range of intelligence. Everyone can learn to be more intelligent, some just have to study and work at it harder. This is when motivation is all important."

The big question is, why are some people highly motivated and others not motivated at all? Some cultures seem to highly motivate its members, whereas other cultures don't seem to motivate its members at all. In many cases, the more normal and contented one is, the less motivated one is. As a rule, those searching for love and approval are the most motivated and highest achievers of all. In my view the most motivated of all are insecure individuals with a need to love or be loved.

"Rufus," said Leroy, "will you do me a favor? Ask me if I care, it's all nonsense." Rufus didn't reply as he turned the Silverado into the bowling alley parking lot.

Inside the bowling alley, Rufus and Leroy greeted the other players who were waiting on their arrival. Their team managed to beat the Harrington All-stars, one of the toughest teams in the league. After saying good-by to two of the younger players, Danny Hebert and Freddie Lee Jr. Brenda Johnson, the nurse and only female member of the team, walked with him and Leroy back to his truck.

Saying good-by to Brenda, Rufus then dropped Leroy off and headed home to Janet. Once home and showered Rufus climbed into bed. "Are you awake Janet?" said Rufus.   s ease

"Yes Rufus, I was just about to doze off, but I am fully awake now." They snuggled together in each others arms, gently kissing and anticipating, but not rushing to that distance, slowly approaching, then faster, still faster explosive ecstasy.

When Rufus arrived at the Harlem

Garden Restaurant the following morning, he could hardly believe his eyes. Someone had scrawled racial graffiti all over his building. After he got inside Rufus immediately called Lt. Elder. He was told Lt. Elder didn't get in until 8 a.m., but he would get in touch soon as he arrived.

Rufus was back in the kitchen preparing breakfast when the phone ring about eight fifteen. "Harlem Garden Restaurant," said Rufus.

"This is Lt. Elder, may I speak to Mr. Thomas?"

"This is he."

"I got a message you wanted me to get in touch with you?"

"Yes, I wanted to report that last night somebody scrawled racial graffiti all over my building."

"Mr. Thomas, most likely it was that same gang that did the drive by shooting. Mr. Thomas give me a couple of days; I'm going to step up the effort. I promise you I'm going to find that gang and bring them to justice."

"I sure hope you find them soon," said Rufus.

"Mr. Thomas, I'll let you know the minute anything turns up." After Lt. Elder hung up, Rufus decided to call his friend Leroy Jackson. The phone rang about three times, then a female voice said,

"Hello."

"Hello Pat. This is Rufus. Is Leroy in?"

"Yes, he's out back. Hold on, I'll go get him."

After about a minute a male voice said, "Hello."

"Hello Leroy, this is Rufus, how are you today?"

"I'm doing pretty good, I was out back doing some work on my lawn mower."

"That damn gang struck again last night," said Rufus.

"What happen?" d she

"They spray painted and scrawled racial graffiti all over my building."

"That's terrible," said Leroy.

"I called Lt. Elder, and he promised me he was going to step up the effort and catch this gang and bring them to justice."

"I know you will be glad," said Leroy.

"You know Leroy, I've already written one letter to the editor, and I'm going to write another one today."

"Rufus, do you really think it will make any difference?"

"Leroy, I think it will. I'm saying things that somebody needs to say about all of this big government and the welfare state."

"Ain't nothing going to change," said Leroy.

"Leroy, I believe somebody must speak out on the destruction that is being done to this country. I've decided to write a book about the dangers of the welfare state and social spending."

"Who are you going to get to publish

it?" asked Leroy.

"I don't know, I may have to publish it myself.   By the way Leroy, "would you like to go fishing with me this Saturday evening at Grassy Pond?"

"Yes, I don't have any other plans."

"Good, I'll leave the restaurant early and let Erica and Zaporia close up. Leroy, I see some customers coming in, got to go now, I will talk to you later."

CHAPTER 6

LaTonya couldn't wait to get home to watch her favorite soap opera, "As The Earth Spins." She had helped her aunt Regina at her cafe all morning. She knew Bruce was probably playing basketball most of the day at one of the basketball courts in the Jimmy Carroll Housing Projects.

A dilemma was haunting her on whether to tell Bruce that Boom Boom had made a pass at her. Boom Boom had come on to her that morning at Regina's Cafe. Boom Boom had told her that he didn't know what she saw in Bruce; why didn't she give a real man a chance. Like himself. She told Boom Boom she wouldn't have anything to do with him if he was the last man on earth.

She knew if she told Bruce there would be a fight or even worse. She prided herself on being able to handle men. She reasoned that unless Boom Boom became too persistent or started harassing her, she would just keep quiet on the whole matter. She had told Bruce that she should be home by two o'clock

       After playing basketball most of the day, Bruce checked his Timex. It was two thirty; he figured LaTonya should be home by now. He told his teammates that would be his last game. Bruce said farewell to the guys and left walking to LaTonya's house. Bruce thought back to last Monday night. He would like to scare the old stooge that runs the Harlem Garden Restaurant off that property, but he didn't want to kill him. He had decided to spray paint the racial graffiti on that building to keep up the pressure. With the neighborhoods changing all around a lot of the older business owners had already been scared off because of the high crime rate. He still believed that with enough pressure, the Harlem Garden Restaurant owner would pull out too.

       As LaTonya's house came into view, Bruce thought LaTonya was a nice catch. Even with two kids, she almost graduated from high school. She often talked about getting her high school G.E.D. Bruce was sure she was going to do it too. He had made it to the tenth grade, but by all practical means he had quit school.

       Being only sixteen, he couldn't marry her now even if she would agree to marry him. He had nothing to offer her.   He couldn't take care of her. He felt fortunate because he was sure LaTonya loved him. He felt some way, somehow he would someday marry her. He would buy her a car, jewelry, furs and other nice things. She was about five eight and weighted around one hundred and forty lbs. with a superb figure. She was very neat and clean. She tried to hide it, but he knew secretly she was very ambitious.

He knew she would never stay on welfare very long. Deep down, Bruce sometimes wondered why she put up with him.   He decided she really did love him. Bruce smiled as he reached out to ring her door bell. He noticed one of the curtains being pulled to one side, immediately after that, LaTonya opened the door. "Hello, LaTonya," said Bruce.

"Hello, Bruce, are you doing all right today."

" I'm doing pretty good." LaTonya stood to the side as Bruce strode into the living room. He sat on the sofa and LaTonya came over and sat beside him. Bruce gave her a long French style kiss. "How did your day go, LaTonya."

"It went okay, how about yours?"

"I played basketball in the projects most of the day."

"Bruce, your mother thinks you are attending school. Good as you play basketball, you should go to school and play on the varsity. I'm sure you could get a scholarship to go to college."

"I don't know, LaTonya," said Bruce.

"Bruce, I've already started studying for my high school G.E.D. I hope to test before the end of the year, and if I pass I plan to enroll at Buieville Community College around the first of next year. I plan on getting my L.P.N. Degree." Bruce leaned over and started French kissing her. Between kisses she whispered to Bruce, "My mother is keeping the kids, we have the whole afternoon to ourselves."

Friday morning Lt. Elder had planned on staying in his office and catching up on his paper work. Around eight thirty, his secretary, Carolyn Laverne, brought him a list of all the cars that had been stolen and recovered within the last two weeks. On the list was a gray Honda Accord. He immediately picked up the phone and dialed Captain Eric Boyd, in charge of the Traffic Division.

"Hello, this is Captain Boyd Traffic Division."

"Eric, this is Marvin Elder over in the Youth Gang Division. I need some information on a gray Honda Accord that was stolen and recovered last week."

"Sure Marvin, I remember the car.   We lifted several sets of fingerprints of that car.

Let me transfer you to Mrs. Veronica Register, she will give you all the information we have on it."

"Hello, this is Mrs. Register, may I help you?"

"Yes, this is Lt. Elder over in Youth Gang Division. I need some information on a gray Honda Accord that was stolen and recovered last week."

"Just a minute, Lt., I need to bring up that file on the computer. Okay what do you need to know?"

"First, I would like to know where was it stolen from." "It was stolen from Eugene Sharpe's used car lot."

"Where was it found."

"It was found on Sirmans' Drive near the Jimmy Carroll Housing Projects."

"Thank you very much, Veronica, I believe that's all I will need. Hold it," said Lt. Elder, "just one last thing, do you know who found the car?"

"Yes, a young patrolman named Douglas Roosevelt on the graveyard shift. That's Captain Anthony Fuller's shift."

"I'm sure that will do it, Veronica, have a nice weekend."

"Same to you Lt." After hanging up, Lt. Elder thought about where the car was found. In almost all cases wherever a stolen car is found, the culprit or culprits live in that general area. He would ask his information sources the names of all gangs operating in and around the Jimmy Carroll Housing

Projects. Lt. Elder decided instead of waiting until Monday he would go down to the Jimmy Carroll Housing Projects and see own to if he could find Littlejohn.

He knew Littlejohn could give him a list of the gangs operating in that area. He grabbed his portable and decided to leave for the Jimmy Carroll Housing Projects. "Carolyn;" said Lt. Elder to his secretary, "I shouldn't be out of the office very long, I'm going out to the Jimmy Carroll Housing Projects."

"Yes sir."

"I have my portable with me in case I have to be located in an emergency."

"Yes sir."

When Lt. Elder arrived at the projects he decided to park near the office building as usual.   He was hoping since it was before noon Littlejohn would still be home. He walked up to Littlejohn's front door and gave about three knocks.   After a few seconds he heard movement inside.

"Who is it?" came a voice from inside.

"Lt. Elder."

"Just a minute." After what seemed like a full minute, Littlejohn opened the door.

Lt. Elder strode past him into the living room. "Littlejohn, I was hoping you would be in, I won't take but a few minutes of your time."

"Okay," said Littlejohn.

"Littlejohn, I have reason to believe the gang I am looking for is in this area." Lt.

Elder got out his notepad and said,

"Littlejohn, I need the names of every gang operating in this area."

"There is a Latin gang, but I can't remember its name. There is the Young Vipers, and a little farther south is the Bonehead gang."

"How about the other gang the Young Vipers?"

"The Young Vipers are mostly kids Lt. Some of them are as young as twelve or thirteen. The leader Bruce Allen is real mean, but seems to have some honor about himself. The real   valueless one is his second in command Boom Boom. Boom Boom is the type that will take both your money and your life and feel no remorse." Lt. Elder reached into his left pocket and pulled out a clip of bills, slid off five twenties and thanked Littlejohn.

"One other thing Littlejohn, where can I find Bruce Allen and the other leaders. Where do they hang out?"

Littlejohn thought for a minute. "Lt. there are two places Bruce Allen likes to hang out. Almost everyday, sometimes during the day, you will find him playing basketball on one of the courts here in the projects. The other place he like to hang out at is, Regina's Cafe down on S. Mary Alice Ave."
On his way back to his office Lt. Elder decided he would wait until Monday to follow up on those names. He believed one of those gangs was the one he was looking for.

Saturday, Rufus told Erica to close up the restaurant. He was taking off early to go fishing. At home, Rufus was deciding on what gear and fishing equipment to use. He decided to take along his spinning reel just in case the biting was slow. Then he might decide to do a little casting for bass using plastic worms. But today, he planned on fishing for bream or blue gill, a very good pan fish.

Rufus decided to use a light limber eight-foot long bamboo cane pole. That would allow him very good wrist action to pitch his bait from spot to spot while the boat slowly trolled the lake. The minute he got a bite, he would quietly anchor down. If he didn't continue getting bites, he would start back trolling. He decided on a number five blue steel hook that would bend without breaking.

He also decided to use a fifteen pound test line with a B.B. shot lead weight, about six inches from the hook and use a small slim line cork so there would be very little resistance when the fish bit and pulled on the hook. He also decided he would take along both crickets and red wigglers for bait. Finally, making sure there were at least two safety vests on board, he decided to give the fifteen foot bass master one last going over.

Then he hooked her up to the Silverado.

Before leaving his house, he called Leroy to let him know that he was on his way. After leaving Leroy's house, they pulled into Alfred Myers Bait and Tackle Shop. They each purchased about fifty crickets and a small container of red wigglers. Now, finally, they were on their way. As he turned   into the Old Stockton Road leading out of the city, Rufus smiled to himself and wondered if Sarah Whitlock still lived on this road.

He remembered years ago she was his first employee at the Harlem Garden Restaurant. She fell in love and married a rich undertaker, then he made her quit to take care of their eventually ten kids. They used to live in a nice colonial style home with bay windows on this road. He watched Leroy light up and take a long drag on his cigarette.

He often thanked God he found the strength several years ago to quit that costly stupid health snatching habit. But he guessed we all have a weakness for something.

"Leroy," said Rufus, "what do you think about people always complaining that they can't find any jobs?

"I don't think there are very many good jobs left," said Leroy, "all we got is jobs flipping hamburgers or some other minimum wage job.

"What I really think," said Rufus," is all of this crying about no jobs is a red herring or some other phony excuse. Just think about it, we have millions of illegal aliens in this country easily finding work. But somehow, poor Americans can't find work. The availability of hard, tough work is the bait that is drawing the illegals to this country. If it was not for our welfare state, those now on welfare would have to do hard tough work, and there would be no jobs left to draw millions of illegals to this country. As for those minimum wage jobs, I have worked them and feel that anyone that has to work will take any job he can get until he can do better. One other thing is, this complaining about rich people making money. Attack the rich is the first thing a dictator or socialist does. They try to falsely blame the rich for all shortcomings. That way they can distract and mislead the uninformed, while they promote their own power grabbing agenda. Balance is the key. we need a strong middle class. Nobody poor is going to give anybody a job, so it stands to reason the more rich people we have and produce the more jobs we all will have. You can't get blood out of a turnip. Somebody has to have money to pay those that don't have any, otherwise nobody will have money to pay those that don't have any, like in a socialist system."

   "Rufus," said Leroy, "don't miss your turn, next right."

   "Okay, I won't. Let me say this last thing and I'll get off this subject. There is no shame in doing hard, tough work as long as one has the freedom and opportunity to better himself. But we will never get Americans to do hard, tough work as long as we have a welfare state like ours. There will always be some excuse not to work."

As they were pulling up to Grassy Pond, Leroy said, "I sure hope we catch a big mess of fish. There is nothing better on a Saturday night than a big bowl of cheese grits, coleslaw, sliced onions, deep fried fish, and hush puppies." Once they got the fourteen foot bass master unloaded, they decided to slowly troll around the east side of the lake first. They decided to start off using cricket first. Rufus took the front seat. He positioned the foot pedal for comfort to best guide and direct the boat. As the bass master named Yvette slowly eased through the water, Rufus used a slight wrist action with his light eight foot pole to pitch his cricket from one spot to the next.

They were about a hundred yards out in the lake when all of a sudden a blue gill hit his bait so hard his bamboo cane pole bent almost to the breaking point. As Rufus finally snatched the blue gill out of the water and let the fish slowly swing back to his open left palm, he then eased it into the live-well.

One of the challenges of bringing in a big blue gill is they will turn sideways on you, then a pound and a half fish will pull like an five pound bass. "Leroy," said Rufus softly, "ease out the anchor." When Rufus snatched the blue gill out of the   water, he saw a clear, watery liquid streaming from the fish. He knew instantly this was their lucky day.

He realized it must be a full moon and the fish were on bed, meaning the fish would be in large groups and the males would be fertilizing the female eggs. He knew if it was a big bed they could catch their allotted amount in short order, because on a bed, you can catch them as fast as you can bait up. Unfortunately, it was a small bed.

They caught about ten blue gills as fast as they could throw out. Then nothing for the next fifteen minutes. It was not long before they found another bed. After being on the pond for a little over two hours, they had their allotted catch, then they headed for home. Once Rufus had dropped Leroy and his share of the fish off, he eased the Silverado back into traffic for the twenty minute drive to his home.

As the Silverado droned on, Rufus thought back to when he was a young petty officer in the U.S. Navy stationed in San Diego. Their daughter Freddy Mae was born after he and Janet had been married a little over a year. Both parents doted on their only daughter. She was taught to be responsible for her actions. She was taught to treat all people well and decently as she would like to be treated no matter how she was treated in return, but always defend herself and not take any abuse. She was taught to always look for a reason to succeed instead of accepting any excuse for failure.

His mind came back to the present as Debra Marie Drive loomed into view. As he turned onto Debra Marie Drive, Rufus smiled to himself and decided he would call his daughter when he got home. Rufus put away his boat and secured everything. He decided to clean just enough fish for a good meal. The rest of the fish he placed in two one gallon plastic milk containers with the top cut off them. He then filled them with water, and placed them in the freezer. He would clean the rest later as needed.

That night, he and Janet enjoyed a supper of cheese grits, cole slaw, sliced raw onions, dill pickle, deep fried fish, and hush puppies. Afterwards, they cuddled together on the sofa in the den, and viewed one of the latest video movies.

"By the way, Janet," said Rufus, "I have managed to finish writing two chapters in my book. I have also decided on a name for it. The name will be "Why We Must Dismantle The Welfare State," by Rufus Thomas.

CHAPTER 7

LaTonya yelled at her two-year-old son because he was making too much noise banging a toy upside the wall. For Christ sake, she couldn't hear what Karen Parker was saying on her favorite soap opera, "As The Earth Spins." She checked the time, it was almost noon. So she decided to boil some wieners. Her boyfriend Bruce should be over soon and he might be hungry.

That reminded her to check her food stamps; the baby was almost out of milk. She would get Bruce to run to the store and get some milk and fruit loops. She put the wieners on slow cooking and returned to the sofa to watch her soap. As she watched the beautiful Earlene Ford seduce her leading man on the "Youth And The Reckless," she thought back to a couple of years ago when her stepfather had tried to rape her.

She had to go live in Miss Louise Gardner's Orphanage for young girls. Miss Gardner was very strict, but she was fair. She taught her girls to believe in themselves, that they could be whatever they wanted to be. Someone knocking on her front door brought her back to the present. LaTonya walked over to the window and slightly parted the curtains to see who it was.

It was Bruce, and she immediately opened the door.

"Hello, LaTonya," said Bruce. "Hello Bruce, how are you today?"

"Pretty good," said Bruce as he strode past her and sat on the living room sofa.

Bruce sat beside her on the sofa. He still found it hard to believe that he could hold on to a charming girl like LaTonya.

"Bruce," said LaTonya, "would you like for me to fix you a couple of hot dogs?"

"Yes, I would like a couple of hot dogs." LaTonya got up walked over to the refrigerator and took   out about three hot dog buns.

"Bruce, what would you like on your hot dogs?"

"Just ketchup and mustard will be fine." LaTonya finished fixing the hot dogs and brought them and a soda to Bruce on the sofa. "Bruce, when you finish eating I would like for you to go to the store and get me some milk, and fruit loops for the kids."

"Okay, LaTonya, I'm going to leave early today. My mom told me to be home when she got off from work. She wants to have a very important talk with me." After finishing up eating   his hot dogs, Bruce left for the nearest Flash Food Minute Market about a block away.

It took him about thirty minutes to return from the minute market. LaTonya made her two kids take their daily nap, then she took Bruce's hand and gently led him to her bedroom. Later, as they lay talking she asked Bruce to please get out of the gang and go back to school. Bruce said he would think about it. Bruce checked his Timex. "LaTonya," said Bruce, "it is almost five o'clock I really must go. I will try to come over later tonight."

"Okay, I will get up and walk you to the door." When Bruce got home, his two sisters, Tasha age fifteen and Tameka age fourteen were doing their homework. His mom was in the bathroom. Bruce sat on the living room sofa and started watching TV. After about fifteen minutes, Bruce's mother Miss Gracie Bell Allen came out of the bathroom.

"Tasha," yelled Ms. Gracie Bell, "is Bruce home yet?"

"Yes maam, he's watching TV in the living room."

"Bruce," yelled Miss Gracie Bell, "I want to talk to you in your room."

"Yes maam." As Bruce ascended the stairs to his room, he wonders what it was that his mother wanted to talk to him about that seemed so important.

He decided to himself that the jig was up; he was busted. He knew it had to be about him playing hooky from school. As his mother stood by his room door, he strode past her into his room and sat on the side of his bed. His mother followed him into the room and closed the door. "Bruce," said Miss Gracie Bell, "I want the truth I don't want to hear any lies. I want to know have you been going to school every morning when you leave here?" Bruce thought about lying but sensed that his mother already knew the truth. After taking longer than necessary to answer, Bruce finally said, "no maam."

"Where have you been going every school day."

"I've been playing basketball here in the projects and going to a friend's house."

"Who is this friend that you have been going to his house instead of going to school?"

"It is a she."

"I see," said his mom. "What is her name?"

"LaTonya Smith."

"How old is she?"

"She just turned eighteen."

"I want to find out more about this LaTonya woman, but that can wait. It was late when you got home last night, and I decided to wait until I got off work today to talk to you. The high school principal's office called me yesterday afternoon, and we had a long talk concerning you. They think you are headed for serious trouble. They think you not only skip school, but you are also involved in gang activity. They feel it is only a matter of time before you will be dealing hard drugs. Bruce, I brought you into this world, and damn it, I will take you out of it. Bruce I have made my share of mistakes, but I will not stand for this. I promise you if you stay in this house, you are going to school. Tomorrow, I'm going out to the school and talk to the principal. I'm going to tell her the first day of school you miss I want to know about it. I may have to send you to live in the country on your uncle Hoover Charles' farm, but you can rest assured that if you skip school again there will be severe consequences. Do you understand me, young man?"

"Yes maam."

Monday morning Lt. Elder had already decided to bring in the leaders of two gangs. He decided to go after the Young Vipers first. The leaders of the Young Vipers were a sixteen- year-old name Bruce Allen, and another sixteen-year-old that went by the name Boom Boom. Lt. Elder knew he may need extra help in making this bust just in case things turned sour. Lt. Elder decided two other sergeants in the youth gang division may not be enough manpower.

He decided to bring in four additional uniformed officers for back up. One of the uniformed officers was a tough battle scarred chap named Lt. Joe Walsh. The other uniformed officers were Staff Sergeant Roger Miller, Corporal Dana Mitchell, and Corporal Charlie Johnson. Lt. Elder had the names of the gang leaders, but he didn't have the slightest idea how these kids looked.

He already had his task force organized and ready to move, but since he didn't know how these kids looked he needed to do a little leg work first. He had already gotten permission from Police Chief Jimmy Sampson to exempt members of his task force from other duties. The Young Vipers were reported to hang out at Regina's Cafe.

Lt. Elder told his secretary to log him out to Regina's Cafe and from there to the Jimmy Carroll Housing Projects. He should be back in a couple of hours. It was around nine thirty when Lt. Elder entered Regina's

Cafe. There were no customers around at the time. The cooking area was behind the counter and about midway behind the counter, was a big, black eight burner gas stove with a large, smooth iron grill on the left and a large baking oven on the right.

At the far end of the counter toward the back of the diner, was what looked to be a storage room and office. Two women, who looked to be in their early thirties, seemed to ignore him and continued with their chores. Clearing his throat, Lt. Elder said, "I would like to speak to the owner."

"I am," said the lady nearest to him with a pleasant voice and ready smile as she turned around to face him. "I'm Miss Felicia Regina, owner of this establishment."

"I'm Lt. Elder from Buieville P.D." as he flashed his badge.

"Miss Regina do you know a sixteen-year-old by the name of Bruce Allen?" I have information that he and his friends come in here often."

Miss Regina looked in the direction of her employee, Miss Anna Ruth Leonard. "Anna Ruth, ain't that the name of the young man that be talking to my niece?"

"I do believe it is, Miss Regina."

"Lt. I do believe I know the young man, what he done?"

"We just need to ask him some questions," said Lt. Elder.

"How about the name Boom Boom; do you know him?"

"I don't think so." "

"Well, he's Bruce Allen's right hand man and is with him most of the time."

"You're right Lt.; the same one or two friends are with him almost all the time."

"Miss Regina, do you have a phone in the back where there is privacy."

"Yes, I have one back in my office."

"Miss Regina, I would like to ask a favor of you. You don't have to do it if you don't want to."

Lt. Elder reached in his shirt pocket and pulled out a card.

"This is the number you can reach me," he said as he handed Miss Regina his card. "I would like for you to give me a call if Bruce Allen or any of his friends come in here today. Remember you don't have to do this if you don't want to."

"I'll give you a call Lt."

"Make sure you use the phone in back because the call must be in complete privacy. Also, make sure you describe the color and type of clothes they are wearing. Before I go, may I use your phone?"

"Sure Lt., come on around behind the counter," as she led him back to her office. Lt. Elder called his secretary and told her to contact him immediately on his portable if he got a call from Regina's Cafe. It was almost ten thirty when Lt. Elder arrived at the Jimmy Carroll Housing Projects.

He parked in the office parking lot as usual and made his way to Littlejohn's apartment. Once inside Littlejohn's apartment, Lt. Elder asked him if he could identify Bruce Allen and Boom Boom.

"Sure, I can identify both of them," said Littlejohn. "I see Bruce Allen playing basketball here in the projects almost every day. Boom Boom don't care as much for basketball, but he do be on the side line watching most of the time."

"What I would like for you to do, Littlejohn, is monitor all of the basketball courts here in the projects and the minute Bruce Allen or Boom Boom shows up give me a call. Since I don't know how he looks, make sure you give a good description of the color and type of clothes they will be wearing." Lt. Elder reached in his shirt pocket and pulled out one of his cards, then reached in his left trouser pocket and pulled out a money clip, slid off a couple of twenties and thanked Littlejohn. Lt. Elder returned to his office and decided to catch up on his paper work while he wait on the expected calls.

It was almost one o'clock when Lt. Elder received the call from Regina's Cafe. Miss Regina told Lt. Elder that two of Bruce Allen's friends were in her place of business. They both looked to be around age sixteen and had on long shirts about three sizes too large. One of the shirts was gray with sea shell like designs, the other shirt was green with flowery designs.

"Okay guys," said Lt. Elder. "Let's go make this bust."

Lt. Elder and the other two plain cloths detectives from the Youth Gang Division rode in his unmarked sedan. Lt. Joe Walsh and the other three uniformed officers rode in two black and whites. Their instructions upon arrival was for the detectives to go in first and the uniformed officers to lag behind a little.

When Lt. Elder pushed open the front door, he immediately spotted the two gang members. He cautiously approached their table and came to a stop directly in front of them. "Buieville P.D.," said Lt. Elder as he flashed his badge.

"Which one of you goes by the name of Boom Boom?"

"I do," said the youth in the gray shirt.

"I'm placing both of you under arrest for suspicion in a driveby shooting. You have the right to remain silent. Anything you say can and will be used against you in a court of law. You have the right to talk to a lawyer and have him present with you while you are being questioned. If you   cannot afford to hire a lawyer one will be appointed to represent you before any questioning, if you wish one. Stand up, turn around, and place your hands behind your back." The two youths did as they was told and showed no resistance.

Both suspects were led outside and placed in one of the black and whites. Lt. Elder dismissed the other two sergeants from the Youth Gang Division plus one black and white and two corporals. He instructed Lt. Joe Walsh and the other uniformed officer in the black and white with the suspects to follow him. He wanted to stop by the Harlem Garden Restaurant on S. Mary Alice Ave.

About ten minutes after leaving Regina's Cafe, they arrived at the Harlem Garden Restaurant. After entering the restaurant, Lt. Elder asked the waitress out front to speak to Mr. Thomas. The waitress went to the kitchen, and Mr. Thomas immediately came out front. "Hello, Lt.," said Mr. Thomas, "what can I do for you?"

"I have a couple of suspects to that driveby shooting outside and I would like for you to see if they were the youths you ran off your parking lot."

"I would be glad to take a look." Lt. Elder led Mr. Thomas out to the black and white. Mr. Thomas leaned over to get a better view of the youths inside. Then he walked a few feet away with Lt. Elder at his side. "The one in the gray shirt was definitely one of the kids I ran off my parking lot."

"Thank you, Mr. Thomas, we will take it from here." Lt. Elder took both youths back to the station for questioning. Boom Boom was told his fingerprints were found on the stolen car, but he denied any involvement in any driveby shooting. He was sent to the district youth correction center in Belview, then two weeks later, he was sentenced to 4 months of boot camp. The other youth broke down during questioning and told everything and was released into the custody of his parents.

CHAPTER 8

Rufus decided he was not going to write a large book and that he would keep it down to around a hundred pages. He estimated he would be finished with his first draft in about another week. Since he identified one of the gang members for Lt. Elder, he felt finally this gang threat would soon be over. He was in a good mood so he decided to do some writing on his manuscript.

He decided to write about one subject that he was truly sick and tired of. He was sick and tired of all this damn blaming everything and everybody but one's self in today's society. You can talk to anyone successful, and they all will tell you the key to success is to try and keep trying no matter the circumstances. People that are always looking for something or somebody to blame are in his view irresponsible and dangerous. Just think about it, he thought, if one is independent and responsible he is not going waste time blaming and depending on others. The surest proof of one's dependency and irresponsibility is wasting time and exercising in futility because someone don't like or accept him. It is irresponsible to waste time blaming others because they don't like you.

The fact is, if you are a good and decent person, good and   decent people are going to accept you, otherwise they don't matter. Who cares so long as they can't hurt you. You can't make people like you if they don't want to, and it's dumb and shallow to think otherwise. The same people that are always blaming others are not doing a damn thing of substance for themselves or their fellow man.

All these years of welfare and social spending have conditioned far too many people to expect the government and others to do for them while they sit back and blame and complain. It has given far too many people a dependent mentality. They feel they are entitled to everything anybody else has without having to earn it. They try to blame and lay a guilt trip on others that prosper and earn their way instead of making their own actions produce worthy results.   It's a matter of focus. When a good ball team gets a bad call, it doesn't start focusing on the officiating but instead keeps its focus on its winning game plan. That is the same way it should be when dealing with racism. One should keep his focus on his goal and not lose focus on racism or anything negative. It's impossible for racist, or haters to destroy your mind unless you hate them back, then your own hate may end up consuming your mind and soul. If you get down into the gutter to settle a dispute with someone, there is no way to come out looking sparkling clean.

Sure, there is racism in this country, and I've faced it first hand, but my focus is on becoming as physically independent and self sufficient as possible. I for one don't fear racism because this country still offers me many options to become as good or successful as anyone. I'm not soft on racism.

I am completely against racism and bigotry in any form. It's just that we live in a real world and it is not wise to completely ignore human nature. The fact is, as long as different races are living among one another there is going to be some racism whether people admit it or not. Many of those complaining the loudest about racism are the biggest racist of them all. It is short sighted for a minority race to be perceived or treated special in anyway, because it divides and turns other races against them. Things like affirmative action and hate crimes on the surface may seem helpful, but in the long run they divides and causes resentment among the races. Sure, big government can protect us now, but nothing remains the same, and sooner or later the majority race is going to get its redress.

Racism will never keep a do-for-yourself person down when he has the freedom and opportunity like in this country. All it is is another obstacle to overcome and overcoming obstacles is what makes successful people successful. The sensible thing is to concede racism, because as long as there are different races one will have to deal with it sooner or later. Whether it is admitted or not, every race has its share of racists.

The solution is instead of all this blaming, we need more do- for-yourself Americans like in the days before the welfare state began. A do-for-yourself person is going to be more concerned about what he is going to do for himself than what somebody else may or may not do.

One other thing, when the liberals keep chanting let's put children first, let's put children first, let's put children first, they forget about the unborn aborted children. They were our future children too. To claim the government is responsible for our children is the main reason why our society is in a complete decline. Every individual parent is solely responsible for his or her own children, not the government , nor anyone else, unless the children are legally taken from the parent. This whole government and society is on the brink of going bankrupt and breaking up like the former Soviet Union unless something is done to save our currency from becoming worthless from out of control spending. Still, you have shallow minded liberals demagoging the issue by hiding behind children. The sad fact is, if we don't start cutting spending and save this great nation nobody is going to be able to help the children or anybody. Sure, liberals care greatly about this nation and the things they advocate, but in most cases, their care is shallow and superficial.

Sixty years ago almost everyone was conservative because of the hardships and struggles to survive. Now, far too many people have become shallow with weak survival instincts, due to big government and social spending. It's a perception problem. You can't get most people to see the value of self sufficiency and tough love in today's society. But, the facts are self sufficiency and tough love are survival tools that could save millions of lives if a severe calamity hit, and believe me, with the decline of our family and moral values this nation is becoming more and more vulnerable. The best thing for a liberal is a little hardship and struggle that will wake him up and open his eyes. A little hardship and struggle will give a liberal some depth by sharpening his survival instinct. A weak survival instinct is why any society that has it too easy, will eventually destroy itself. There has to be some real, or imposed hardship and struggle in one's life in order to build good judgment and character.

Rufus checked his watch; it was well

after five, so he decided he had better quit writing for now. He closed up the restaurant and went on home. On Friday nights, Rufus and Janet liked to attend all of their local high school home football games. Tonight, the Buieville Tigers were playing cross town rival, Hutto High Trojans at home.

It was around seven thirty on this clear fall night when Rufus and Janet left for the game. The sleek, new Towncar cruised through the silent, crisp cool South Georgia night air with the smooth grace of a champion race horse. They arrived at Lomax Field about ten to eight. That would give them ten minutes to settle in their seats before game time.

Tonight, the Buieville Tigers were facing undefeated cross town arch rival Hutto High Trojans. At half-time, the Tigers were up fourteen to seven. Late in the fourth quarter, the Tigers were down twenty to twenty-one with only fifteen seconds left in the game. On second and goal, the Tigers had just taken their last time out with the ball on the Hutto High Trojans' two yard line. Instead of kicking a field goal it appears the Tigers are going to run another play.

The referee windmills his hand to signal that time has started. The Tigers all state quarterback Hoover Sirmans II is under center. He drops straight back about five yards, he looks, he looks, he looks, ten, nine, eight, seven, six, all receivers covered Sirmans zooms the ball over everyone's head out the back of the end zone. Three seconds left on the clock, the kicking team automatically runs onto the field. Both teams are set. The kick holder gives the signal. The hike is good. The kick holder places the ball. The soccer style kicker follows through and keeps his head down, never looking up until he hears the roar of the crowd, then he is literally mobbed. There is sheer pandemonium as the home crowd goes wild.

Rufus still felt elated as he and Janet left the stadium and headed for home. "Janet," said Rufus, "I feel like celebrating a little, how about us stopping by the Dairy Queen for some ice cream?" "That would be nice, Rufus, I believe I will have a banana split." There was no line so Rufus was able to drive straight up to the drive-in station.

"May I help you?" said the speaker at the drive-in station.

"Give me a large cup of ice cream with nuts on top and a banana split," said Rufus.

"Will that be all sir?"

"Yes."

"That will be three seventy five, drive around please."

Rufus received his order, paid his bill, and headed for home. After arriving home, Rufus and Janet sat on the sofa in the den. Rufus put on some soft oldies music and they enjoyed their ice cream. Later they fell asleep in each other's arms after consummating the night in perfect bliss and ecstasy.

CHAPTER 9

Around three thirty, Lt. Elder and the other officers were still on alert static. "Lt. Elder, Littlejohn on line two," said his secretary Carolyn Laverne.

"Lt. Elder speaking."

"Lt. I have bad news, I can't figure it out, Bruce Allen is always playing basketball everyday here in the projects. I don't know what happened, but I haven't seen him all day."

"Littlejohn," said Lt. Elder, "you can call it a day.   I appreciate the effort you gave it."

After hanging up from talking to Littlejohn, Lt. Elder decided he was going to release most of the task force. He decided to hold over two of the uniformed officers, Lt. Joe Walsh and Corporal Dana Mitchell. Everyone else was dismissed. During questioning, they managed to get some crucial information out of the youth with Boom Boom.

They know where Bruce Allen lives, where he supposedly went to school, where his girl friend lives, etc. After releasing the other members of the task force, Lt. Elder in his sedan and the two uniformed officers in their black and white, headed for Bruce

Allen's home in the Jimmy Carroll Housing Projects. It was after four o'clock when they arrived at Bruce Allen's address.

Lt. Elder and the other two uniform officers walked up to Bruce Allen's apartment. Lt. Elder pulled the screen door back and gave three loud raps.

"Who is it?" said someone from the inside.

"The police."

A wide eyed girl opened the door immediately.

" Does Bruce Allen live here?" said Lt. Elder.

"Yes sir."

"We would like to talk to him."

"He ain't home."

"Do you know where we can find him?"

"No sir."

As Lt. Elder and the officers walked back to their cars, "Joe," said Lt. Elder, "school has already turned out for the day. The most likely place he will be is at his girl friend's house."

Shortly thereafter they arrived at LaTonya's home on Cummings Street. As the officer's approached LaTonya's front door, Lt. Elder instructed Corporal Mitchell to go around to the back door just in case Bruce tried to skip out. When Lt. Elder knocked on the front door, they noticed a curtain near the door part slightly. Within a few seconds, a young lady opened the door about eight inches.

Past her, Lt. Elder could see a young man sitting on the sofa.

"Is Bruce Allen here," said Lt. Elder?

The young lady just stared at him for several seconds. Finally, she said,

"Yes, he is here."

"We would like to talk to him." LaTonya opened the door wide and stood aside. Lt. Elder and Lt. Joe Walsh entered the living room.

"Are you Bruce Allen?" said Lt. Elder to the young man sitting on the sofa.

"Yes sir, I am," said Bruce Allen.

"I am placing you under arrest as a suspect in a driveby shooting. You have the right to remain silent. Anything you say can and will be used against you in a court of law. You have the right to talk to a lawyer and have him present with you while you are being questioned. If you cannot afford to hire a lawyer one will be appointed to represent you before any questioning, if you wish one. Stand up, turn around, and place your hands behind your back." Bruce Allen did as he was told and offered no resistance.

Lt. Elder used his car phone to call Rufus Thomas at the Harlem Garden Restaurant, but he didn't get an answer. He then called Mr. Thomas' home and his wife said he hadn't arrived from the restaurant yet. Lt. Elder left word for Mr. Thomas to call him at his office as soon as he got home. Back at the station, Lt. Elder questioned Bruce Allen about his involvement in the driveby shooting on the Harlem Garden Restaurant.

Bruce Allen denied any involvement in the drive by shooting or the spraying of graffiti. Around five thirty, Rufus Thomas called. Lt. Elder asked him if he would come down and identify another youth that he believed was involved in the driveby shooting. Mr. Thomas said he would be there in about thirty minutes. Lt. Elder also called Bruce Allen's mother and informed her of the trouble Bruce was in. She said she would be down right away.

Upon arrival at the station, Rufus Thomas told the desk sergeant why he was there. The desk sergeant paged Lt. Elder to the front desk. "I'm glad you could come down, Mr. Thomas," said Lt. Elder as he approached the front desk.

"I'm more than glad to do whatever I can to help bring these criminals to justice."

"Come with me, Mr. Thomas," said Lt. Elder as he led him to a viewing room that was behind a two way mirror.

Once inside the viewing room, Lt. Elder told Mr. Thomas to see if the youth in the other room was one of the youths he ran off his property.

"That's him," said Mr. Thomas, "that's the one that did the talking."

"Are you absolutely sure," said Lt. Elder.

"Without a doubt in my mind."

"Thank you very much, Mr. Thomas,

you can go now."

Lt. Elder led him back to the front desk. "Thanks again, Mr. Thomas, for coming."

"You're welcome."

After Mr. Thomas' departure, Lt. Elder begin making arrangements to have Bruce Allen transported to the district youth correction center at Belview. Lt. Elder was paged to the front desk. He was sure it must be Miss Gracie Bell Allen, Bruce Allen's mother. "Hello, I'm Lt. Elder. Are you, Bruce Allen's mother?" asked Lt. Elder as he approached the front desk.

"Yes, I'm his mother."

"Miss Allen, we are sure your son is guilty. We have a witness and your son's fingerprints were found on the stolen car that was used in the driveby shooting. We cannot turn him loose in your custody. This evening he will be taken to the district youth correction center at Belview. Then in about two weeks he will go before a judge. Since this is his first arrest, the judge will probably sentence him to four months of boot camp instead of him facing a jury trial and receiving time in an adult prison. Come with me Miss Allen, you will be allowed a thirty minute visit."

After Miss Allen left and all arrangements had been made to transport Bruce Allen to Belview, Lt. Elder decided to go home; he still had time to make it to the Buieville High Tigers football game.

Rufus took his spiritual life very seriously. Serving the Lord was a well established tradition in his family. His uncle was a preacher, and his father was a deacon. He also had a brother who was a minister and two other brothers who were deacons.

Growing up, Rufus didn't have a choice about going to church. His father's law was, "me and my family will serve the Lord." As a young man, Rufus had sowed his share of wild oats, but even when young he had the sense to never experiment with drugs. Otherwise, he stayed out late, partied hard, and did a lot of things he shouldn't have. Old Prospect Baptist Church was the family church.

As young as he could remember as a boy, he had sat in the pews of the Old Prospect Baptist Church. While away in the navy he sort of backslid from his religious upbringing. Even back home out of the navy it was several years before he started back attending church regularly. Then about ten years ago, he became a deacon at Old Prospect Baptist Church. He also has been a Sunday school teacher almost as long.

On Sunday mornings, Rufus liked for Janet to fix him one of those old fashioned southern country breakfasts. She would fix homemade buttermilk biscuits, smoked sausage, Canadian bacon, grits, scrambled eggs, jelly, real butter, and orange juice.

After breakfast, they left for Sunday school. Their regular pastor would not be preaching today. Today's guest speaker would be visiting pastor Rev. John B. Miley.

After the eleven o'clock service had started and Rev. Miley launched into his sermon, Rufus' mind drifted back to some of the great sermons his late cousin Rev. Robert Flagler of Fernandina Beach Florida used to preach. He remembered how Rev. Flagler stressed Philippians fourth chapter, thirteen verse, "I can do all things through Christ who strengthens me." He stressed how anyone down and out with little or no self confidence could repeat that verse over and over to themselves at least fifty times a day, and it would guarantee them a successful life if only they kept saying it. Here is another good   positive saying to repeat fifty times or more each day to help one lose weight, "I'm going to have a slim body, soon." The mind tries to fulfill any image constantly presented to it. It doesn't matter whether it is real or imagined, positive or negative. The mind doesn't distinguish; it only recognizes images. That is why it is so important to think positive. That is why many of the old sayings have grains of truth in them, sayings like, "Out of sight out of mind," this can be a factor concerning sex education, and a scary man can't win in gambling or in battle.

The mind can't remember and deal with all of our experience at once, so it tends to remember and act on the images that is presented the most constantly. The images that are presented less and less will soon be forgotten and not acted upon, but like in everything there are exceptions. For instance, in cases of trauma, an indelible imprint can be stamped in one's memory in a matter of seconds and last forever.

Another old saying used when someone was struggling with a problem was, "Go home and sleep on it." There is great benefit in that because it allows the subconscious mind time to help sort out and organize the problem. The mind receives so many conflicting images during a day that one would go crazy if the mind didn't use sleeping and dreaming as a sorting and filing process to organize recent images. Most of us are not aware of the negative thought images that we constantly feed our mind, but the good thing is we can make a conscious effort to think of positive images.

We have the ability to choose. One can decide how he will treat another human being no matter how that person treats him in return. The most powerful positive thinking image I know of is to love and forgive all people no matter how they treat you.
That doesn't mean you let anybody mistreat you. You always defend yourself from attacks. You can hate a person's ways and actions but still love the person as a human being.

There may be cases when someone is

determined to make them, you hate them, then turn it over to God, just repeat to yourself,

" I can wish all people goodwill even if it's not returned." When you treat other people well, and they don't return the favor, you are not doing them a favor; you are doing yourself a favor, because as long as you treat all people well, you will stay a good person and mostly good things will happen in your life.   Then nothing nor anybody can mentally defeat or destroy you.

You never see those who can genuinely love and forgive in mental wards, you won't see them as bums on the streets, or losers in any way. It is not enough to say I don't hate anybody, what really matters is how things are acted out. That means how you actually treat all people on a day-to-day basis. There is no way you can hate anybody, not even your enemy if you make it a practice to treat all people well like you would a loved one.

Sure, there is a need for hate and all emotions, but never hate anybody in your midst unless you are prepared and able to destroy them, lest they destroy you. The rule of thumb is to choose to treat all people well with courtesy and respect. When Rev. Miley's voice roared into one of those soul stirring hymns, it brought Rufus' mind back to the present.

After the service, Rev. Miley stood at the front door and shook the hands of the congregation as they filed out. In the

Towncar on their way to Mitchell's Barbecue Restaurant for their Sunday dinner, Janet asked Rufus how he liked the sermon Rev. Miley preached.

"Rev. Miley preached a great sermon," said Rufus, "but to be frank I spent most of the time remembering some of the great sermons my late cousin Robert Flagler used to preach. My view on religion is I believe in God as much as anyone, but I also believes God helps those who first help themselves.

I believe if you do as good as you can do or go as far as you can go, then some way, somehow God will help you go the distance. Otherwise faith without action is wasted." They had a nice Sunday dinner of southern fried chicken, barbecue ribs, mustard greens, potato salad, macaroni and cheese, rice and gravy, sweet potato pie, corn bread, and iced tea.

Once back home Rufus decided to send out several queries to find a publisher for his almost completed book.

CHAPTER 10

Bruce Allen had never seen his mother as angry and upset as when she found out he had not been going to school. No matter how much he thought that going to school was a waste of time, he knew he didn't have any choice because his mother was dead serious. The next day at school he felt out of place, but he knew he had to make the best of a bad situation. Somehow, he got through his first day back.

He felt especially elated when the bell ring ended the school day. Not so much because school was letting out but because he was going to see LaTonya. He and LaTonya were watching TV when they heard someone knocking on her front door. When Bruce heard someone ask for him with an unmistaken tone of authority, he knew instantly it was the police and he knew why they were there.

He knew it was too late to go out the back door because they had already seen him sitting on the couch. He knew there was no point in trying to resist, he might as well go quietly. After being arrested and taken to the station, he was fingerprinted and booked. During questioning, he denied having anything to do with any driveby shooting. They claimed they lifted his fingerprints off of a gray Honda Accord that had been stolen the night of the drive by shooting.

Lt. Elder repeatedly asked him if he was in anyway involved in a driveby shooting. Each time they asked, he denied everything. Later, what bothered him most was the pain and hurt in his mother's eyes. He felt he had truly let his mother down. He loved his mother more than life itself. He decided then and there that if he ever got through this trouble he would swear before God to go straight, because never again would he put his mother through that kind of hurt and pain.

After he had told his mother how sorry he was for having told hurt her, he then told her if the Lord got him through this, he would finish school and leave gangs and drugs behind. With tears in his eyes, he told his mother good by. Sergeant Victory Kocher, a young detective on the night shift, transported him the thirty miles to the district youth correction center at Belview.

At the center he was issued brogans, coveralls, underwear, tooth paste and tooth brush, and bed linen. The next morning he had to meet with the center's chief psychiatrist Doctor Zebedee Moore, then he had an appointment with the center's rehabilitated strong man, Chaplain David Taylor. He was assigned to dormitory "B." Each dorm was managed by a supervisor.

He was to report to his dorm supervisor any problems or criticism he had. He was told he would be there until his court date in about two weeks. Bruce was not used to being told every thing to do, in fact he had never had any strict discipline, period. He managed to adjust to the regimental style of life better than he at first imagined. He had been at the center now for almost two weeks, and his court date would be coming up in a few days.

It's been almost two weeks now since Lt. Elder put those youth gang leaders behind bars. Rufus felt good about how his life was going at the present. Business was good at the restaurant. The gang problem had been taken care of. He had   found a publisher for his book. So he decided he would celebrate by buying Janet a diamond ring.

Lee's Press, Inc. a small publishing company would be publishing his first book. The small publishing company couldn't promote it as much as Rufus knew it deserved, so he knew if the book was going to make it big he would have to do a lot of the promoting himself. He would try to get on the Frances Waddell talk show and as many talk shows as possible.

The publishing company was going to start off with sixty thousand copies for the first printing. They will give him two hundred copies to give to friends, do self-promoting, sell or do as he pleased. The publisher was going to run some ads in a few big city newspapers, but Rufus knew that for the book to sell he would have to make the rounds of talk shows and hustle his own book.

Juvenile Judge Fred Smith had very

little sympathy for spoiled, ill-raised, undisciplined youngsters. He felt lack of discipline was the root cause of all the problems with today's youths. Most of the kids that come before him have never been conditioned to fear punishment or consequences. Many of these kids have never heard a cold hard firm voice of authority demanding obedience. They look at him wide-eyed and bewildered when he chews them out.

Judge Smith knew that most of the kids that come before him would never be there if someone would have shown them love and put the fear of punishment and consequences in them the first time they broke the law. Most of the people running around talking about people being mean spirited are too shallow to see past their noses. They are hollering that conservatives don't have any compassion. They don't know what real compassion is. Real compassion is about protecting and saving the whole country, not about saving a few and letting the whole country perish and go to hell.

We all have a free will to adapt, but to waste compassion on those that choose not to adapt is not only a waste of time, it is dangerous. All animal or specie survival is dependent on their ability to adapt to their environment, otherwise they perish. Not forcing people to depend on themselves, their family, their extended family, their community, and private organizations is being weak, irresponsible, and negligent, not showing compassion. It is always easier to be weak and take the course of least resistance, but in the end it will cost this country dearly if not destroy it. Real compassion is to be prepared to survive as an organized society under all conditions, even if the government goes broke and money becomes worthless. Trying to get liberals to understand that is like talking to a brick wall. Those with the foresight and wisdom must speak out on the necessity of conditioning people to depend on each other as much as possible for their survival. No one knows how much time we have to prepare, but the destruction of moral and family values are always the last stage. Big government is the cause of the problem, not the answer.

Judge Smith knew he could save more of these youngsters if he could put the fear of God in them, thereby conditioning them to fear punishment and consequences.

Bruce didn't know what to expect as he sat in juvenile court that Monday morning when his name was called. His mother was sitting on his left, and uniformed officer corporal Andrew Desantis was on his right. After his name was called, Officer Desantis escorted him to a rail about ten feet in front of the judge then left him alone and stood off to one side.

As Bruce stood there, the judge continued to read a report.

"State your name," said Judge Smith to Bruce in a loud, demanding voice.

"Bruce Allen, your honor" (as he had been coached).

"How do you plead to the charges?" said Judge Smith.

"Not guilty, your honor."

"We have an eye witness, and how did your fingerprints get on a stolen car that was believed to be used in the driveby shooting?"

"I don't know, your honor."

"Young man, you could go before a jury and be sentenced to several years of hard time in prison as an adult, but since this is the first time you have come before me, I am going to sentence you to four months of boot camp at Pine Valley Youth Correction Institution. But if you ever come before me again young man you are going to be put away for a long, long time. Do you hear me young man," said Judge Smith in a loud cold angry voice.

"Yes sir your honor."

"Take him away, bailiff," said Judge Smith. Bruce was allowed to say good bye to his mother and LaTonya. Then he was taken to boot camp at Pine Valley Correction Institution.

At Pine Valley every thing was done in regimental style like in a real military boot camp. After arriving at Pine Valley, he was issued clothing and assigned a bunk in an open bay dormitory. Every morning they had to get up at five thirty. They were given thirty minutes to make their beds with perfect hospital corners, brush their teeth, shave, shower, etc.. Breakfast was served from six to seven.

Calisthenics was from seven to nine. Classes and training were from nine to twelve. Lunch from twelve to one. Classes and training from one to four thirty. Dinner from four thirty to five thirty. Recreation and leisure time from five thirty to ten p.m.. At ten p.m. all lights out. Bruce was taught to say yes sir or no sir to every command or instruction. Some of the training instructors were retired military.

One of his instructors was a mean tough, computer whiz named Sergeant Johnnie Roberson. Bruce remembers his first morning at reveille. They had to stand at attention while Sergeant Roberson walked up and down the line inspecting the prisoners. He stopped in front of Bruce and placed his face about four inches from his. "What is your name prisoner?" said Sergeant Roberson in a loud, angry voice.

"Bruce Allen sir."

"I can't hear you."

"Bruce Allen, sir," said he in a loud voice.

"I still can't hear you."

"Bruce Allen sir," said he almost yelling.

"Where you from prisoner?"

"Buieville, Georgia sir."

"The only thing that comes from there is skunks and punks, which one are you prisoner?"

"Neither, sir."

"Are you calling me a liar prisoner?"

"No sir."

"I'm going to be watching you prisoner, and if I see you step out of line, your ass is grass and I'm the lawn mower, do you hear me prisoner?"

"Yes sir."

Sergeant Roberson took several steps backward, then he yelled out, "Column right, hut, two, three, four, hut, two, three, four," and on they marched to the dining hall.

At first, Bruce wanted to rebel and resist being told everything to do, but after a while he learned to control his anger and actions. Then for the first time in his life he felt a new power and control over his actions. He realized one's own actions determines the results one gets out of life. After more than a month at Pine Valley, Bruce knew that he was going to make it. He had gained enough self-control to do the right thing and stay out of trouble.

His mother and LaTonya visited and stood by him.   The least he could do would be to stay out of trouble and not let them down.

CHAPTER 11

It's been almost a week since Rufus received his free two hundred copies of his first book, "Why We Must Dismantle The Welfare State By Rufus Thomas." Rufus had immediately started doing his share to promote his new book. He sent copies to all of the major book suppliers around the country. He sent copies to all of the largest big city newspapers. He also sent copies to major public and college library systems around the country.

He requested to be on several talk shows. He offered to lecture and sign copies of his book at public functions, churches, prisons, etc. Within the next three months, he had invitations to appear on the Frances Waddell talk show and several other talk shows. Next month he was scheduled to speak at Pine Valley Youth Correction Institution.

Rufus had no intention of ever seeking public office himself, but if he could convince just one person in office of the dangers of big government and the welfare state, that alone would make it all worthwhile. The government has taken on a provider role and is saddled with huge financial burdens with millions and millions of people, some totally dependent on the government for their only survival. That is irresponsible and negligent for any free society to do; this especially when the government doesn't have the self-discipline to control spending. What are all those people to do when the government go broke. Only a fool will believe it can't happen.

It is obvious that it is only a matter of time before the debt gets so big the government can't raise taxes high enough, borrow enough money, or sell enough bonds to finance it. Then the government won't have any choice but to print more and more money. After a while printing all of this money will cause hyper-inflation making the greenback practically worthless. With a very weak nuclear family and extended family system this country could lose fifty million plus people and split along regional and ethnic lines. With our loose family and moral values there is no solid foundation left to organize and rebuild upon. With money being worthless, there would be nothing the government could do without international help. But if the dollar went down, it would probably bring the world economy down with it. The economy is already so distorted that our currency is like monopoly money with the way sports figures and entertainers are being paid.

What are we to do, with the family and the extended family structure almost destroyed from fifty years of becoming dependent on an over generous, non-disciplining, and super rich sugar daddy government. On the other hand, when responsibility is passed to the states and local governments that should help rebuild the family foundation, then if the central government went broke, all would not be lost. One month later Rufus was up, up, thirty three thousand feet into "the long, delirious burning blue," The wild blue yonder,"Where never lark, or even eagle flew," on his way to the Big Apple to appear on the Frances Waddell talk show. It was an all expense paid trip.

On the show, Rufus was asked how can you be so uncaring as to cut out school children's lunch program money? We have to ask ourselves this question, said Rufus, which is more   important, to cause much hardship or lose the whole country. I say save the country first, then the children may have to take a lunch pail or bag to school or whatever is necessary. People will always find a way to survive on their own unless they depend on the government so long and forget how to do for themselves.

After returning to Buieville, Rufus enjoyed his new fame. He and his book received a big write up in the "Buieville Daily Times." His publisher reported that his book was selling great. At the rate they were selling, the initial sixty thousand would be sold out in two weeks. The publisher was already making preparations for a second printing.

Three weeks later Rufus spoke at Pine Valley Youth Correction Institution. Afterward he signed copies of his new book. As Rufus was signing books he was surprised and taken aback when Bruce Allen wanted Rufus to sign a book for him. Rufus thought of his religious upbringing, he thought of a youth gone astray, and he thought of the power of forgiveness. Rufus stared at the young man.

"Mr. Thomas," said Bruce Allen, "I'm sure you know who I am."

"I do?"

"If you find it in your heart to forgive me of the wrong I've done you, I just want you to know that I'm truly sorry."

"What are you going to do when you get out?" said Rufus.

"I promised my mom that I would finish school, sir."

Rufus thought that a young man living with his family in the Jimmy Carroll Housing Projects could use some pocket spending money. "I'll tell you what young man, if you are willing to work, come to see me at the restaurant when you get out." That night Rufus lay relaxing in bed after he and Janet had made love. "You know Janet," said Rufus "a strange thing happened to me today at my speaking engagement at Pine Valley Correction Institution. One of the youths convicted in the drive by shooting on my restaurant bought one of my books and wanted me to sign it. He told me he was sorry about what he had done. I not only autographed his book, I offered him a job when he gets out, but I can't help but wonder if I did a dumb thing."

"Honey, you've always enjoyed helping people.   You wouldn't be happy any other way."

"I guess you're right, dear. Good night, darling," said Rufus.

CHAPTER 12

After four months, Bruce had done his time and was let out of boot camp, but he still was on probation for another four years. Bruce was determined to keep his promise to his mom. He decided to stay away from his old friends and the gang. He decided no matter what, he was going to finish school. He got word that Boom Boom had become leader of the Young Vipers. Bruce tried out for the Buieville High basketball team.   He not only made the team, he was going to be a starter.

His girl friend LaTonya had passed her high school G.E.D. and was scheduled to enroll at Buieville Community College the next quarter to get her L.P.N. Degree. Three weeks later, Bruce and LaTonya were watching TV when the newscaster reported that a local gang leader who went by the name of Boom Boom was killed last night in a driveby shooting.

A few nights later Bruce was sitting with LaTonya on the sofa. "You know, LaTonya," said Bruce, "I stopped by the funeral home this afternoon to see Boom Boom, and deep down in my soul, I knew that the body lying there could just as easily have been me. Truly the Lord does work in mysterious ways," said Bruce. "At the time I thought being arrested was the worst thing that could have happened to me, but as it turned out being arrested and going to boot camp was actually the very best thing to ever happen to me. It gave me a second chance to live, and I'm going to make the best of it. Boom Boom blew his second chance, but not me."

"Honey, I am so proud of you," said LaTonya.

"Thank you dear, but I could never have done it without you and mom's support."

Rufus was back in the kitchen when Erica stuck her head in the doorway. "Mr. Thomas, there is a young man out here that says he would like to talk with you."

"Erica, tell him I'll be there in a minute." As Rufus pushed open the kitchen door he recognized the young man as Bruce Allen immediately. Rufus walked behind the counter to right across from where Bruce Allen was standing.

"Hello, Mr. Thomas," said Bruce Allen as Rufus came to a stop.

"Hello Bruce."

"Mr. Thomas, I came by to see if you are still willing to give me a job."

" We close around three thirty during the week, but we stay open to nine p.m. on

Friday and Saturdays, so I can let you come in for a twelve hour day on Saturday if you would like that."

"Yes sir, Mr. Thomas. I certainly would appreciate it."

"When would you like to start?"

"Quick as I can; this Saturday will be fine."

"Fine," said Rufus, "I will pay you minimum wage; be here at eight a.m. this Saturday."

"Yes sir, I'll be here, and thank you very much Mr. Thomas."

Rufus knew about fifty dollars wasn't a lot of money, but it would help teach the youth the work ethic and provide him with pocket money. After four Saturdays Bruce proved to be a dependable, willing worker. Rufus and Bruce sort of took to each other. Rufus never had a son and Bruce never had a dad; it seemed to be a perfect match. Already, Rufus had taken Bruce fishing in his boat, the first time Bruce had ever been fishing in his life.

Detective Marvin Elder stopped by the restaurant often to chat a few minutes and have a cup of coffee with Rufus. Rufus' book had gone into its second printing. He couldn't judge how much effect his book had to do with the mood of the country, but he took comfort in observing the whole country going through a peaceful revolution. Even the bleeding heart liberals were admitting something had to be done about the welfare

mess. Only in the U.S. can a poor, shy
country boy rise up and touch the heartbeat
of America. Rufus decided to end his book
by saying, God bless America.
THE END

**Self-made writer Freddie L.
Sirmans, Sr.
Writer/publisher/philosopher/
Inventor.
Website: FLSirmans.com**